Health And
Happiness

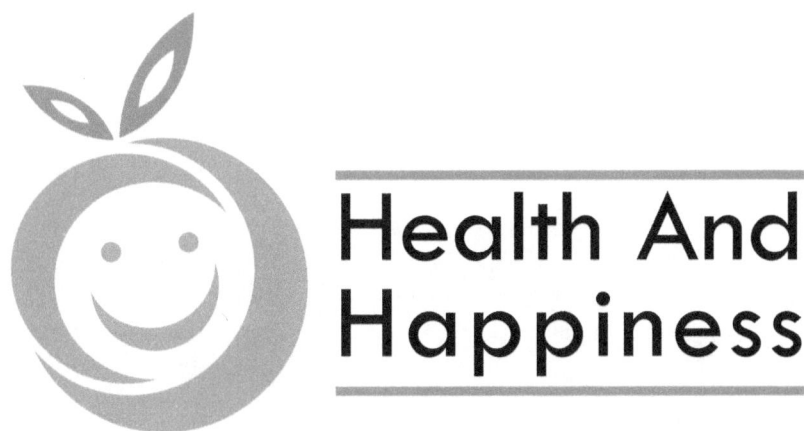

Health And Happiness

Sean Donovan

"an owner's manual for the mind and body"

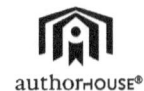

authorHOUSE®

AuthorHouse™
1663 Liberty Drive
Bloomington, IN 47403
www.authorhouse.com
Phone: 1-800-839-8640

First published by AuthorHouse   1/14/2010

ISBN: 978-1-4490-6602-4 (e)
ISBN: 978-1-4490-6600-0 (sc)
ISBN: 978-1-4490-6601-7 (hc)

Library of Congress Control Number: 2010900187

Printed in the United States of America
Bloomington, Indiana

This book is printed on acid-free paper.

Table of Contents

Dedication

THIS BOOK IS DEDICATED TO the millions and millions of good people who have met untimely deaths due to cancer and disease that could have and should have been prevented. This book is dedicated in their memory to the billions of people who are still alive but have been affected by the loss of their loved ones.

This book is dedicated to the millions of cancer survivors and chronically ill who have survived their challenges and fought to live another day. Take your second chance and run with it. Live life to its fullest and appreciate every day as if you should have died yesterday. I hope my book may shed some light on possible reasons why you were "chosen" to fight your battle. I hope the information and technologies in this book may help prevent you from ever having to go through another ordeal like that again.

This book is dedicated to the millions of people who are overweight and don't want to be, but don't know what to do to make permanent changes that will affect their weight, health, lives and attitude. I will explain how a fork can be a "weapon of mass destruction".

This book is also dedicated to the smokers, drinkers and drug addicts who want to quit but can't seem to find the willpower and stick-to-itiveness to make the change and stick to it.

This book is dedicated to anyone who is depressed – whether they know it or not. Every day spent in a fog of depression – void of smiles, laughter, love, self worth, positivity and mental clarity is a day not lived to its fullest and a day that can never be replaced.

This book is dedicated to the healthy, happy people who already know and practice all of the information contained herein. Good for you! I hope this book will help reinforce the things you already know and encourage you to keep up the good work. Maybe it will even inspire you or motivate you to influence someone else to make a change in their lives too. If you fight for health and prevention every day before you have a problem – you may never have one. If you wait until you have a diagnosis of a terminal illness – it may be too late.

This book is dedicated to worldwide health reform – both mental and physical. This book is my contribution to the well being of others. I believe everyone should give back to the community and this is my repayment to society for all of the good fortunes I have had in my life. Certain people have taken the time and interest in me and shared some valuable health and life advice that I would like to now pass on to everyone. Plus – I believe that if you are healthy and happy you will be able to return the favor to me one day with a simple smile.

"Focus on what you can control and the rest will fall into place. Start with your attitude because it is the one thing that you truly have 100% control over."

Introduction

HEALTH REFORM IS CURRENTLY THE single most important change that we, as a society, must achieve. Time is of the essence because every day thousands lose their health insurance, millions get ill and countless preventable deaths happen daily. Health, along with time, is paramount and should be held at the top of our priority list. Neither health nor time can be replaced or purchased once they are gone. Both must be appreciated and used to their maximum in the moment they are present. Without health everything else is irrelevant – when you are dead, dying or sick it is tough to enjoy life. Everyone should care about their health regardless of age, race, sex, religion, national origin, career, or income level. We all have only one body and one chance at life. We all have the same 24 hours in a day, but there are no guarantees on how many days each of us will have.

Health reform is so important that the President of the USA has made it his top priority in spite of two ongoing wars, a global economic crisis and all-time unemployment highs. I commend him for recognizing the importance of health reform, but I would like to cut through the red tape and bureaucracy behind it. I am going to break down health reform in a language and terms that everyone can understand without regard to political affiliation, income level or current insurance carrier. This Health and Happiness guide will help lay the foundation for nationwide health reform - one person at a time.

Health reform is both mental and physical. Health reform starts at the "grass roots" level. It starts with the daily decisions that we, both individually and collectively as a society, make regarding our health. Our health depends on whether we decide to eat an apple or a candy bar – drink water or a soda – smoke a cigarette or take a run – pop an aspirin or practice yoga – sit on the couch and watch TV or sit in a park and watch the sunset – shape our faces and form our attitudes with a smile or a frown. These are the daily decisions and choices that we make and have control over. Choosing to make the right ones and actually following through is the key. It all starts with us – the people – at home, at school, at work, in our cars and in our daily lives and routines. So start making the right decisions today. Deciding to read this book is the first step in the right direction.

Let me pose a few questions to you. Are you happy with your mind and body? Do you feel like you perform at 100% all of the time? Could you jump out of your chair right now and go run 2 miles with little effort? Do you smoke? Are you overweight or have just a few pounds you would like to lose? Do you get headaches? How much water do you drink daily? Do you sleep restfully? Does your energy last all day? Do you eat "fast food"? Do you use deodorant? Do you have a history of cancer or heart problems in your family? How long do you think you will live?

If any of the questions I asked concern or interest you… Then take a while to explore this health and happiness guide. You only live once and you only get one body. Be good to yourself and you will last a long time and perform well. Or if you are going to abuse your body – at least give it the tools it needs to repair itself on a regular basis!

Every car, appliance, electronic equipment or tool that you purchase today comes with instructions or an owner's manual. The human body is far more complex than anything money can buy, but unfortunately human beings do not come with a manual or instructions. We must rely on our instincts, the teachings of our parents and those we watch growing up - And oh yeah... commercials, food producers, pharmaceutical companies, "drive-thru doctors" and those who have a monetary interest in our health.

My primary goal is to educate you and open your eyes to a new level of health and a new way of life. Please remember – I am not a doctor, nor do I claim to be. The following guide is a combination of facts, opinions, beliefs, "educated speculation" and common sense. This is my instruction manual for the human body and my recipe for happiness and health. It has worked for me – so keep an open mind and check it out!

Health

WHAT IS HEALTH? HERE IS my definition:
H.E.A.L.T.H – Heightened Energy And Love That Heals.
H.E.A.L – Heightened Energy And Love.

What is heightened energy? I define heightened energy as raising your body's metabolic rate, brain power, awareness, concentration, emotion, activity and energy levels to their maximum potential. Heightened energy is using your body to its fullest capability and performing as close to 100% as possible all of the time.

What is love? Love is a positive emotion that usually equals happiness. Love is an emotional bond with oneself, another person or something else. Love causes positive emotions which causes hormone and endorphin release in the body which causes positive attitude, which reduces stress and leads to more productivity and heightened energy.

What is success? Success is feeling a sense of accomplishment and worth in oneself.

There is a circle between health, happiness, love and success. They all go hand in hand as one leads to the other.

A healthy body is one that is full of positive energy and has a strong immune system with the ability to defend itself from disease and heal itself after injury.

Disease

DIS-EASE: MY DEFINITION OF DISEASE is anything that robs you of your health and happiness.

Some of the top diseases in our society today include:

- Heart disease (Heart attack, high blood pressure) - claims approximately 2700 lives daily in our country

- Cancer (breast, colon, prostate, lung, lymphoma, etc...)

- Stroke

- Autism

- Alzheimer's disease and dementia

- Depression

- HIV (AIDS)

- Irritable Bowel Syndrome (IBS, diarrhea)

- Erectile dysfunction and infertility

- Obesity

- Sleep disorders

- Migraine headaches

There are hundreds, if not thousands more ailments that plague humans today. Although there may not be one specific cause or one specific "cure" for these diseases and conditions, I strongly believe that there are common denominators that contribute to all of our woes. I believe that the cure for disease lies in the prevention and that the key to prevention lies in the daily decisions we make and the lifestyle that we choose to live. Some of us may be prone to more problems than others, therefore necessitating extra care and compensation on their part. We will explore many avenues of prevention and discuss roads leading to disease in this book.

Prevention

PREVENTION = ACTIONS THAT REDUCE exposure or other risks, keep people from getting sick, or keep disease from getting worse.

Prevention is where we are really missing the boat in health reform. It seems like science is stuck on trying to invent drugs and treatments to cure cancer or disease once we get it and that politicians are stuck on improving the 'health care system' by making health insurance and medical treatments available and affordable, but it makes more sense to put the same time, energy, money and focus into things that will prevent getting disease and needing drugs or medical treatment in the first place. We must find a happy medium and balance between medicine, technology and nature.

Why not make it mandatory for people who receive government subsidies for food or health care to visit a gym or community fitness center for "x" number of hours per day or week? Why not give free health seminars or nutritional counseling to the public to coach people about the proper foods to eat and how their bodies work? Why not limit the foods that can be purchased with subsidized programs to only fresh, natural foods? Why not tax candy, sodas, cigarettes and alcohol 400% or more? If a candy bar costs $5 and an apple costs $0.50 or if a can of soda costs $5 and a bottle of water costs $1, maybe that would help motivate people to make smart (and economical choices) about what they eat. If people really want to eat junk food and smoke cigarettes and drink alcohol, then they should have to pay for it in more ways than just compromising their health. Since these things seem to be the culprits causing a lot of our health woes, then the government should use the increased taxes generated from the sale of these products to pay for the health care to treat the diseases that they cause.

Our body has a natural defense system that is supposed to protect us from disease. Our skin is our outer defense and limits what gets into our bodies. Internally, we have beneficial bacteria, white blood cells and other microorganisms which defend our bodies from intruders such as harmful bacteria, viruses and mutant cells. Anti-oxidants are substances that are ingested in our bodies primarily from eating fresh, raw fruits and vegetables. These anti-oxidants neutralize "free radicals" or toxicity in our bodies and promote healthy cells and even slow down or reverse the effects of aging.

To better explain the importance of prevention and maintenance on your body I will use a simple analogy. Imagine you buy a new car. The car has all of the bells and whistles including leather seats, navigation system, performance engine etc... Now imagine the factory that made the car got carried away with all of the extras on the car, but forgot to apply the most important thing to its body - paint. The paint is a vital part of the protection on the car that leads to longevity, performance and good looks. I compare the paint on a car to the anti-oxidants you must constantly add to your body. Cars are constantly exposed to "free radicals" such as rain, snow, ice, bird poop, road debris and the most detrimental thing to metal on a car - oxygen. Oxygen "oxidizes" the metal in a car and causes it to rust much like toxic free radicals in our bodies attack our cells and cause aging, cancer and disease. Without a good paint job, the car would quickly rust on the outside and expose the internal parts to the detrimental elements as well. The leather seats, carpeting, and electronics will deteriorate quicker than the metal body when exposed to rain, sun and other "free radicals". Just as cars are subjected to constant contact with these detrimental elements, our bodies are constantly bombarded by toxins and free radicals from internal and external sources as well. We breathe in pollution, drink chemically treated tap water, eat processed foods, expose our bodies to harmful radiation from external sources, but our bodies also create their own free radicals within from metabolic processes and digestion. That's right - our bodies create toxins that must be eliminated much like a car creates exhaust and heat as byproducts of burning fuel. The cleaner, higher grade of fuel we burn, the cleaner the byproducts and waste should be and the machine will run more efficiently. If we put a low grade of fuel mixed with toxins and impurities into a car, its engine and fuel delivery system will clog up and ultimately break - much like our hearts and blood vessels do when we introduce impurities into our bodies. If we allow our car's air filter to become clogged and don't clean or change it, the engine will gasp for air and suffocate and will be robbed of power and gas mileage - much like smoking does to our lungs, drinking does to our liver and eating unhealthy does to our kidneys. These organs can be cleansed and detoxified with hydration, exercise and the proper diet so the body can regain lost efficiency and power. Routine daily maintenance will prolong the life of your car and your body and allow them to perform at their peak power and efficiency.

Prevention is the key to curing disease. The cure for cancer and disease is clearly not to get it in the first place. Start the fight against disease before it happens and it may never occur. If you wait until symptoms are present, it may be too late.

In this book, you will learn ways to promote prevention and good mental and physical health - starting with the following list of key ingredients of life.

Essential Elements of a Happy, Healthy Life

THESE ARE THE ELEMENTS THAT I feel are crucial ingredients for a happy, healthy life.

1. Fresh, clean, mineral rich **Water**

2. Fresh, clean, pollution free **Air**

3. Direct **Sunlight** (in the right proportion at the right times)

4. Nutrient-rich, raw, organic **Nutritious Food**

5. Restful **Sleep** and **Relaxation**

6. **Passion** about something you love (a hobby, music, special interests etc…)

7. **Love** and emotional stability with family and friends

8. **Success** and a feeling of self-worth and contribution

9. **Positivity** and attitude control

10. **Exercise,** mobility and movement

You Only Live Once

Is IT POSSIBLE THAT ONE person could smoke cigarettes all of their lives and live to be 100 years old while someone else who never smoked could develop lung cancer simply from breathing in toxic vapors from the out-gassing of the materials in the interior of their new car? It doesn't seem logical or fair, but my father told me at a young age that life isn't always fair. The following story is a prime example of just how unfair life can be.

No matter what you do with your life, never forget that there will only be one now. If you are not happy – change it quickly. We are only here for a flash. Time is definitely the most valuable asset we have. You should have control over how you spend your time and you should always maintain total control over your attitude and emotions. Even if you are incarcerated behind bars, you may not have control over your physical location, but you can still maintain your mind and thoughts. "Focus on what you can control and the rest will fall into place. Start with your attitude because it is the one thing that you truly have 100% control over."

If your house burns down, you can look at it negatively or positively. You could spend your life lamenting over lost possessions or you can thank your lucky stars that you were not lost in the fire too. You may have lost all of your material possessions and the roof over your head, but remind yourself that it could have been worse. Don't let the fire burn the smile off of your face.

If a loved one dies or leaves you, be thankful that you had that person in your life for the time that you did. Carry on their energy and legacy in your everyday life. Let their spirit drive and motivate you to do and carry out all of the good things that they did regularly. Let their soul live vicariously through you. Go out and do all of the things they didn't have time to do before they died. Learn from the goodness of those in your life whether they are dead or alive and thrive on their positive energy.

Avoid negativity like the plague. You become like your surroundings so choose them wisely. Do your best to bring positivity to friends and family in their times of need, but avoid people who are constantly negative and drain your positivity. You probably know who I am talking about. There is probably someone you know who constantly complains, who is never happy or satisfied, but does nothing about it other than complain. You may feel as if they constantly rain on your parade. Get a big umbrella and shield yourself from that person!

In my opinion, there are 3 types of people in the world. The first type of person is someone who is inherently happy, strives to be their best, succeed, love, prosper and help as many other people as they can along the way. The second type of person is someone who may "waffle" between happiness and misery – confused about their own feelings and emotions. They are often jealous and may strive to do better just to outdo someone else while hurting others along the way. The third type of person is one that is inherently unhappy. They find happiness in their own misery and the misfortune and pain of others. Often this person is afraid of success and will sabotage themselves and others just to gain comfort in the negative state of misery that they have come to know.

I would like to share a story about a very influential woman who is at the top of my list of positive people. She changed my life in so many positive ways. Unfortunately, she will never know how much of an impact she had on me because most of her influence occurred on her death bed. Her name was Kathleen and she worked for me as a property manager and leasing agent for over a year. Kathleen was in her mid thirties and was full of spirit and positive energy. She was always the first one in the office in the morning and she was guaranteed to have a smile on her face no matter what was going on. Everyone she worked with and customers she dealt with were always very complimentary of her attitude and work ethic. At times, she may not have had the sales volume of the other agents because of the amount of time and effort she put into one-on-one service with her customers. As a sales manager, I recognized this and called it the "Kathleen Factor" which I applied to her sales quota with a grain of salt. I could always count on her to complete every deal in the most professional manner from beginning to end. She was very competitive, but only with herself.

She worked for me for almost a year before divulging that she was a breast cancer survivor. Over 5 years prior, she was diagnosed with advanced breast cancer and, after a double mastectomy and extensive radiation and chemo-therapy, her cancer went into full remission. For 5 years she got a clean bill of health from her doctor. She told me in a conversation that she felt like she was "living on borrowed time" and wanted to make the best of every moment of it. I can't help but think that it was her positive attitude that helped pull her through the cancer in the first place.

Everything was just fine and dandy in her life until one morning when she came into the office limping. I noticed it at the morning sales meeting and immediately questioned her condition. She shrugged it off and said she just had a stiff hip joint – "must have slept on it funny" she said. She carried on her normal routine all day showing third floor apartments, climbing steps, walking and getting in and out of her car. By the end of the day I could tell she was really struggling, but she insisted she was fine. Judging from the smile still on her face I believed her. The next morning, however, I got a call from her about 30 minutes before work started. She told me that she was going to the emergency room to get her leg checked out. In spite of the fact her leg was now totally paralyzed, she had taken the initiative to call and email all of her appointments for the day and let them know she would have to reschedule. She spent the entire day in the emergency room and was then admitted into a permanent room. When I called to check on her, I knew something was terribly wrong when she did not answer. Another leasing agent and I went to the hospital that night to check on her. After a long wait, we were allowed into her room. She was cheerful and happy to see us and informed us that they were doing some tests to find out what the problem with her leg was and she expected to be back on her feet and back to work in a day or so. I appreciated her high hopes and positive spirit, but quietly knew in my mind that there was a serious problem going on. The three of us chatted and joked for a while and I assured her that all of her clients and appointments would be covered. She expressed concern numerous times about how all of her pending deals should be handled – reiterating to me (her manager) the importance of following up on certain details with each of her clients. Even laid-up in the hospital with sudden, unexplained paralysis in her leg she was genuinely concerned about her clients and my business. Well, I was equally concerned about her and I let her know it in a positive way. When I left with the other agent, we were both silent because no one wanted to state a bad case scenario.

The very next morning, I got a call from Kathleen. With all of my heart I hoped that she would tell me she sprained her hip flexor and was in a leg brace and on her way home. Not the case. She came right out and told me in the most positive and cheerful voice that "I have another battle to fight. Apparently the cancer has returned in an advanced stage in my lymph nodes and has gotten into my spine causing some problems for the nerves in my leg. So I will not be back to work this week".

I didn't know how to respond other than to tell her to forget about work for now. Her response was to remind me again how important it was to her that her clients were handled properly until she returned to work. I assured her they would be and I reported back to her with routine status reports. She spent the next couple of weeks in the hospital receiving various treatments and was then sent home with an around the clock nurse to tend to her since she lived alone. I talked to her frequently, but didn't see her for a week or two. When she told me she was getting discharged from the hospital, she inquired if she could return to work in a limited capacity. Of course, she couldn't drive or climb steps so her position as leasing agent was not possible, but she requested to help out at the reception desk. Our receptionist was more than happy to take over some leasing duties and get out of the office for a while, so I made arrangements for Kathleen to come into work as receptionist the next day. When she showed up the next morning (her usual 30 minutes early) I was stunned, shocked and speechless. No matter how hard it was for me to try to contain my facial expressions and demeanor, it was just not possible. She struggled up the front sidewalk with the aid of her nurse and a walker. If the office had not been closed, I would have thought it was an elderly handicapped customer coming to inquire about property. Every bit of hair on her head was gone. She had nearly doubled in size as if someone had stuck an air hose in her and blown her up like a balloon. Physically, she had almost no resemblance to her previous self – except for one thing – the big smile on her face. I wanted to tell her to go home and lay down, but I knew how excited she was to be coming back to work. Plus, lying down and resting just wasn't in her nature. So I mustered up every bit of positivity I had in my body and did my best to keep a smile on my face as I met her at the door. For the next two days, she sat at the front receptionist desk and answered every call on the first ring and met every customer with a smile. When people inquired about her condition, she had no shame and simply told them that "I am dealing with some challenges". Those two days at work brought her great happiness. She called many of her former customers to follow up and make sure they were happy. By being at work, she brought a whole new positivity to the office and all of the employees.

After two days of working, she became bedridden and was no longer able to function properly. Shortly after that, she was admitted to a hospice center. It took a great deal of motivation for me to go see her in that environment and condition, but I did. I will never forget my last visit with her. My business partner and I stopped by with flowers. She appeared to be half conscious and delirious, but finally recognized us and a big smile formed on her face. The nurse informed us that the cancer had spread rapidly to her brain and that she was losing motor functions and her ability to speak. I told her how much we missed her and wished there was something we could do for her. She began to mutter something to me. I strained to hear her as I bent down closer to her bed. She struggled to form a sentence and keep her thoughts straight, but after a couple of minutes I deciphered what she was saying. She was asking me if she still had a real estate license. That may have been the last time I cried in my life. I suppressed my emotions as best as possible and told her – "Of course you still have a real estate license. It is hanging on the wall in the office waiting for you to return to work." She smiled with satisfaction and said nothing else. Those would be the last words I heard from her. The next day she passed away.

As a real estate broker, it is my responsibility to return all agent licenses to the State Board if an agent leaves my brokerage firm through change in employment or even death. One of the hardest things I ever had to do in my life was to remove her license off of the wall in the office. I made a photo copy of it before sending it back to The Board. I kept the copy of her license on my bulletin board above my desk as a reminder of her. With memories of her came a renewed sense of appreciation of life and people. I strived (as a manager) to live up to her level of customer service on a daily basis. I also dismissed things that used to stress me out and bother me with a "Kathleen style smile."

I will never know what caused her cancer and if she could have done anything to prevent it, but I promised myself one thing – I would share her story with everyone in hopes that it would carry on her energy and legacy by making people smile and appreciate their lives, jobs and health more. It was an unbelievable situation to me – how fast someone's health could deteriorate - yet how positive, happy and caring someone could remain during such an ordeal while facing eminent death. If this story made you cry, dry your eyes, crack a smile and go out and do your best today. You never know when you may wake up with a little pain in your leg.

My Motive

MY NUMBER ONE MOTIVE IS to motivate. I want to motivate you to make positive changes in your life and the lives of others. I truly want to see people healthy and happy – especially those close to me because seeing other people smiling makes me smile too. I want people to live longer, happier lives free from disease, stress and other ailments. I get my happiness from seeing other people happy. There is no greater gift than to make someone smile. So take the knowledge you learn in this reading and pass it along to someone who needs it. Share a smile with a stranger – you may make their day and you may make a new friend along the way.

I am also fed up with our society's outlook on health and disease prevention. I am angry that someone like Kathleen can fight a cancer battle, lose her breasts, irradiate and chemically poison her body with chemotherapy and get a clean bill of health from her doctors - only to have the cancer return 5 years later in a different form and kill her at age 36. She did nothing wrong - she didn't deserve it. She was positive and happy. She loved life. She didn't smoke or drink. What caused her problem - twice? Her doctors never offered any explanations as to what may have caused her cancer(s). Her doctors never dug deep and questioned her personal life including every product she used and food she ate. This was also the case for my other family members who had cancer - their doctors offered up no explanation, solution or possible preventative measures for the future. The only lifestyle question asked by doctors was whether they smoked or not. I think there are a lot of other factors besides smoking that are contributing to the cancer epidemic in our society today. It also stands to reason to me that if you get cancer once, survive, but make no changes in your life - there is a good chance that whatever caused your cancer will remain present and return to haunt you again later. It is my hope that my influence through this book may help prevent someone from having a health crisis. If this book saves only one person's life - then it is a success. If I can make everyone who reads it a little healthier and happier then that is the icing on the cake of life!

If you want or need to change your life – then do it! Appreciate life and live it to the fullest. You only live once – make the most of it. You only get one body – so take care of it. Here is my recipe to get you started on the road to Health and Happiness.

Time is ticking

As I STATED PREVIOUSLY, TIME and health go hand in hand as the two most valuable commodities in the world. Both are far more important than money or any material possession. Although having money does allow you to make better use of your time, it cannot buy time back once it has passed. Money will pay for health care, drugs, vitamins and health food, but health itself cannot be purchased.

Surprisingly, time is one of the top excuses I hear for lack of maintaining health. "I just don't have time in my busy schedule to work out, to grocery shop, to cook and to stretch. I just don't have time after a busy day at work to worry about my lifestyle or to think about my health. I have kids and other responsibilities..." People often say to me.

I challenge you to do a community service exercise that will benefit a total stranger and also help you appreciate time and what you have. Do a good deed and visit a nursing home or hospice care clinic. Find someone who is dying of a terminal illness and sit down and talk to them about time. Imagine yourself lying on your own death bed watching the clock tick – each second bringing you closer to death. I bet you that they have a different appreciation and perspective on time. They probably wish that they had more time or could go back in time and change their health or the way they lived certain aspects of their life. Ironically, every day brings all of us closer to death. Most of us don't think about that until we are diagnosed with a terminal illness. When the doctor says you've got 6 months to live, it puts finality to your life – a date to dread, a countdown to the end of your life. However, don't be a pessimist and look at every day as one less day of life, but rather appreciate every day. Maybe if you did look at each day that way, it would create a greater respect for time.

In the grand scheme of things, there should be nothing more important to spend your time on than your health. You only get one life and one body. Time can never be replaced, so spend it wisely. Every minute that you devote to your health will make your life longer and more enjoyable. When you are healthier and happier, you are able to be more productive and spend more quality time with family and friends. When you take the time to care for yourself, you may prevent friends and family from having to devote a lot of their time to take care of you if you become ill.

The good news is that it is never too late to change how you spend your time (until you are dead).

I think that at least half of every day should be devoted to the most important thing in the world – you and your body. There are 24 hours in a day. 8 hours or 33% of your day should be devoted to sleep, rest and relaxation. 2 ½ hours or 10% of your day should be spent as follows: 1 hour of aerobic activity (walking, running, swimming, biking) to get the heart rate up and the body moving, 30 minutes of anaerobic activity or strenuous aerobic activity (weight lifting, body pump, Pilates, aerobics), 40 minutes of yoga, stretching and meditation, 20 minutes of sauna or "sweat time". Another 1 ½ hours or roughly 7% of your time should be devoted to meal preparation (shopping, cooking, eating and cleaning up). If you follow that formula you will be well rested, thoroughly stretched, exercised, cleansed, well fed and still have 8 hours to work and another 4 hours of extra time. Multi-task and maximize your time even more - stretch while in the sauna, Flexercise while sitting in traffic, prepare several days worth of meals at once.

If you prioritize your life and devote time to the things that really matter the most you will find that the quality of your life will improve and your time will seem more productive and abundant.

One of my favorite quotes comes from James Dean. He said "Dream as if you will live forever, live as if you will die today." To me, that statement shows maximum appreciation for time and life.

Nature is Natural

IMAGINE EVERYTHING MAN-MADE JUST VANISHED. What would the world look like with no buildings or cars or pollution? What would we look like with no clothes, makeup, razors or soap? How would our schedules differ if we had to walk everywhere - and hunt and grow our own food instead of commuting in traffic while eating fast food and irradiating our brains with cell-phone waves? It would be a different world full of different stresses. Catching or picking your next meal would certainly outweigh making it to work on time on the "all natural priority list". Believe it or not this fantasy world still exists in some areas of the world today. We often forget that we came from nature and therefore we are 'all natural'.

Ok, back to reality. Our society has overly domesticated itself and detached itself from nature and natural instincts. Realistically, I doubt hardly anyone (including myself) would be willing to give up all of the creature comforts that we now enjoy. However, what would you be willing to give up if your life depended on it? If you found out that ten years from now you would have a massive brain tumor that would make your last months of life miserable and ultimately claim your life – would you stop using your cell phone today - even if there was only a 5% chance that the phone caused it? Would you eat another fast food hamburger if you knew that next year you would have a massive heart attack and die?

I gave up fast food well over fifteen years ago and never missed it once. I have been a vegetarian for fourteen years and don't crave meat now even though every prior meal consisted of meat and potatoes. I still use my cell phone, but use an earpiece. I quit drinking chemically treated city tap water and drink only the purest mineral rich artesian water imported directly from FIJI. I still drink alcohol on occasion, but try to drink red wine and beer made with natural ingredients and pure water. I drive a gas-guzzling truck, but mostly for work purposes and I keep it well maintained and use the best gas to minimize pollution. I walk or bike for leisure transportation to get both exercise and compensate for my driving. I live by a rigorous and sometimes stressful schedule, so I reward my body with extra relaxation, meditation, chiropractic treatments, yoga, stretching and hot tub time.

My point is that if you can't give up all of the bad things, then compromise and give a lot of good things to your body in return. If you do one bad thing, then counteract it with one or more good things.

Get in touch with nature and your body. Watch stress melt away as you take a stroll in the park on a beautiful day as you breathe in fresh air and listen to birds chirp. Smell the sweet smell of your skin producing vitamin D as the sun's rays beam down onto your body. Feel the energy in the air before a storm, feel the soothing effects of a babbling brook or the hypnotic sound of waves breaking onto a beach. Nature is one of the best stress relievers around.

By getting in touch with nature, you help your mind, body and soul get in touch with itself.

Signatures

SIGNATURES OR "SIGNS OF NATURE" are mother earth's hints to help out where our instincts may be lacking. They can be both warning signs and reward signs. For instance, animals in tune with nature can feel the barometric pressure drop before the coming of a storm and they know that is their signal to take cover. For those animals a little less sensitive, the crack of the first lightning bolt and boom of thunder is sure to get their attention. What does the hiss of a snake, the roar of a lion, the spikes on a porcupine or the aroma of a skunk tell us? – back off! On the flip side, how does the natural attraction to a beautiful flower, a sweet smelling mint leaf or a cute and cuddly bunny rabbit feel?

Less obvious signatures can lead to wonderful health rewards for those who are keen enough to recognize and utilize them. You may have heard that carrots are rich in beta carotene and are excellent for eyesight. Have you noticed that when you cut a cross section of a carrot that (although orange) it looks like the iris of an eye? Walnuts are heralded for their brain stimulation and memory enhancing qualities. Crack one open and guess what – it looks like a brain. Pharmaceutical companies are touting lycopene as a miracle drug for heart disorders. Guess where lycopene comes from – tomatoes! Cut a tomato horizontally and it looks just like a heart – red inside and out, blood-like juice and it even has 4 chambers! How about an avocado? Avocados are rich in magnesium to help your body convert food to energy as well as oils and fatty acids which have been found to be essential in the health of the female reproductive system – especially when pregnant! The pear-shaped avocado looks a lot like a pregnant woman and even has a big pit (seed) in its belly! An avocado even takes 9 months to grow and reach a ripe, edible maturity. Figs look like male testes and guess what - they promote health of the male reproductive organs. Citrus fruits such as oranges and grapefruits look like breasts and have been found to help prevent breast cancer. All of these examples are pretty coincidental signs of nature.

Food for thought: Humans are the only animals on the planet that cook their food. Cooking food cooks out vital nutrients and kills living enzymes in the food.

Eating raw, living foods such as fruits and veggies promotes life. Eating dead food such as meat and things in a box promote death and burial in a box - 6 feet under. When a carnivore in the wild eats meat, it hunts its prey, kills it and then eats it immediately while the flesh is still "alive". A lion doesn't refrigerate, cook or add preservatives to his food - which brings another point. If you look at the digestive system of a carnivore such as a lion you will find that it is very short relative to the animal's body and is an easy straight shot to the "exit". This is to enable the animal to get rid of the waste and toxic by-products formed from digestion of meat. Vegetarian animals have very long and curvaceous digestive systems which retain food for long periods of time to extract everything from the nutrient rich fruits and veggies. Humans have long, curvaceous intestines many times the length of their own bodies concurrent with that of a vegetarian animal.

I believe in evolution and concur that we probably evolved from monkeys - our vegetarian predecessors. I also believe in adaption and survival of the fittest. I think humans were designed to be vegetarians in ideal circumstances, but developed the ability to digest meat during times of drought, famine and ice-age where fruits and vegetables were not available. Now we have over-domesticated ourselves and forced the body to digest chemicals and artificial foods along with meat that was grown, slaughtered and preserved with un-natural feed, antibiotics, steroids, hormones, preservatives and colorings. The side effects are evident today as cancer, heart disease, obesity, autism and numerous other diseases.

Are these signatures just coincidental or is nature trying to tell us something? Unfortunately, so many people have become over-domesticated and completely detached from nature and their senses that we can't see the signs. It is a wonder how we find our way in out of the rain! Speaking of rain... let's move on to water.

We're Water

THE EARTH IS **70%** COVERED by water and your body is supposed to be 70% water. Scientists agree that liquid water is necessary for all forms of life as we know it. In fact water is the one common criterion in their search for extraterrestrial life in the universe.

How much water do you drink? It is my belief that the average American drinks less than 10% of the amount of water their body needs. I think that most people walk around dehydrated on a daily basis. I believe that dehydration is the leading cause of health problems such as obesity, cancer, heart disease and infection. It is also estimated that 85% of all headaches are directly related to dehydration!

My belief can be rationalized and summed up with a simple analogy. Imagine a toilet. There is water in the bowl that you can see and water hidden in the tank waiting to flush. A toilet flush utilizes gravity and hydraulic pressure. There is a balance between the amount of water in the tank, the bowl and the size of the drain pipe. If this balance is disturbed, the toilet won't flush properly. If you removed half of the amount of water in the tank, you would lose flushing power and the waste in the bowl would not disappear down the drain. If you continued adding waste and not enough water, the bowl is going to fill up. Then it's time to get a plunger!

Of course the human body is much more complex than a toilet, but it too needs water to flush waste. The body is basically a system of tubes. These tubes can easily become constricted or clogged with plaque and toxins.

When the tubes become clogged, toxins can't get out and nutrients can't get in. When this happens, swelling and inflammation occur. Inflammation ultimately results in disease.

The body eliminates waste in several forms - through the bowels, urine, sweat and breathing – all of which require water. The lymphatic system is the body's septic system. The body contains six times more lymphatic fluid than blood. The lymphatic system does not have forced flow such as the heart does for the blood or the diaphragm does for the lungs. Rather, the lymph system relies on motion, gravity and water to flow and cleanse itself. The lymph system will stagnate with lack of muscle movement, but the lymph system can benefit from even the smallest motion of the pulsing of blood vessels when heart rate increases during exercise. The body cannot excrete toxins from lymph nodes if you don't sweat or if you seal the toxins in with deodorant/antiperspirant and the lymph system cannot flow and flush itself when the body is dehydrated.

Several things are responsible for lack of sweat - dehydration, lack of exercise and use of deodorant/antiperspirant. Your largest lymph node is in your arm pit. Most Americans use deodorant with antiperspirant sealing the armpit and not allowing it to sweat, thus trapping toxins in the lymphatic system. The lymphatic system connects the lymph nodes all over the body allowing toxins to spread. The most immediate soft tissue area to your armpits is in the breasts. What if one day it is discovered that the leading cause of breast cancer is deodorant and the leading cause of all cancer is dehydration, deodorant and lack of exercise?

The body also needs water to carry nutrients and cool itself. Cells need a clean, nutrient, oxygen and water rich environment to function and multiply properly.

Sweat is a very important bodily function responsible for cooling and cleansing the body. Sweat can be induced by exercise or by spending time in a hot environment such as a sauna. I choose to maximize my sweating each day with rigorous cardiovascular aerobic exercise such as biking or running. After I warm up with the aerobic activity and get the sweat flowing, I then go to anaerobic exercise and lift weights. I then build core strength while stretching and breathing in yoga. I top my workouts off with 20 minutes in the 180 degree sauna. I believe that sweating for

20 minutes in the sauna detoxifies the body more than the kidneys do naturally in a 24 hour period.

Keeping my body hydrated during my workout regimen and my daily activities is vital. My daily nutrient rich mineral water intake ranges from 4 to 6 liters. I know that sounds like a lot – and it is – compared to what most people drink. I drink one liter in the morning within a half hour of waking up. The first meal of the day is known as breakfast – which refers to breaking the fast that your body goes through while sleeping (unless you eat in your sleep). Not only does your body not get any food during the night, but it also doesn't get any water while you sleep. Your body detoxifies during the night by exhaling toxins out in water vapor during your deep, slumbering breaths. Do you ever wake up in the morning with dry mouth and bad breath? Look at your tongue in the morning before you brush your teeth – is it white and dry looking or pink and red and moist? If it looks white and dry, it is toxic and signifies dehydration. A healthy tongue should be moist and red and pink in color. Often, the first thing a doctor will do is pull out your tongue and inspect it – he is looking for dehydration and toxicity. Drink water first thing in the morning and you will feel fresh, clean and energized the rest of the day.

I also drink one liter of water within two hours of sleep each night. Doing this makes it likely that you will have to wake at least once during the night to urinate, but it makes it less likely that you will dehydrate during sleep. During the course of a 90 minute workout I consume another liter of water. Throughout the day, depending on the temperature and my activity level, I will consume another one or two liters of nutrient rich mineral water. My goal is to always have a bottle of water within reach and never let myself get thirsty.

The sixth and most interesting liter of water I consume each day takes place during my 20 minute sauna session. Before I enter the sauna, I strip and weigh myself on a digital scale that has accuracy to a 10th of a pound decimal. I then weigh my one liter bottle of FIJI Water which weighs right at 2 pounds (a gallon of water weighs 8 pounds and there are 3.8 liters in a gallon). My goal is to drink the whole liter of water during the first 10 minutes in the sauna (which is easy to do in 180 degree heat). Then I sweat for an entire twenty minutes. I exit the sauna after 20 minutes, jump in a cool (or cold if you can tolerate it) shower for about a minute and then return to the sauna for about 2 minutes. This hot to cold to hot action essentially wrings out the body much like you do to a wet towel when you twist it up. The sudden shock of the cold shower causes your muscles to tense up and squeeze out lactic acid and toxins into the blood. Returning to the sauna for a couple of minutes then opens up the blood vessels and pores and gets the blood and sweat flowing to carry away these toxins from the muscles they were trapped in. Massaging your muscles (always from limb toward heart) particularly your lymph nodes in your neck, armpit and groin will also help to get toxins moving toward elimination. After my twenty minute sauna experience, I then towel off all of the sweat and water from my body, strip down and weigh myself again. My goal is to weigh the exact same amount as I did when I first entered the sauna before drinking 2 pounds of water. Essentially, I sweat out 2 pounds of water which carries out toxins with it. Some days I weigh more, some days I weigh less, but I usually come within a few tenths of a pound of where I started.

I honestly think that drinking copious amounts of mineral rich water is the single most important thing that you can do for your health. Be leery of municipal tap water that is probably treated with chlorine and fluoride. It is essential that municipal tap water be treated with chlorine to kill harmful bacteria in the water supply - especially when the water supply is recaptured sewer water. The problem with treating water to kill bacteria is that the chemicals in the water cannot discriminate between the bad bacteria and the beneficial bacteria that live in our bodies and carry out bodily functions such as digestion. When these chemicals are ingested into our bodies from tap water, they can wipe out colonies of billions of beneficial bacteria - thus leaving a void in the functionality of the digestive system. This void can be recognized by side effects such as heartburn, indigestion, gas, bloating and diarrhea. Filtered water strips out vital mineral nutrients, but leaves behind chemicals. Avoid cheap bottled water unless you know the source. Cheaper bottled water also tends to have cheaper plastic in the bottle which leaches chemicals out into the water. Don't be afraid to spend a little more money for quality water. I recommend **FIJI Water** which filters through volcanic rock and picks up magnesium, silicates and other minerals. FIJI is also far from industrialized, pollution-producing areas of the world. Another great source is glacial water which is also full of minerals and isolated from pollution.

Drink, sweat, breathe and pee – this will make you toxin free!

Fruits and Veggies

ASIDE FROM DRINKING PLENTY OF pure, clean, mineral rich water, the most important thing you can do to achieve better health is to eat lots of fresh, organic fruits and vegetables. In fact, it is so important to eat fresh, raw fruits and veggies that the National Cancer Institute, American Dietetic Association, American Medical Association, US Food and Drug Administration all recommend incorporating at least 5 servings into your diet daily. Some benefits of eating raw fruits and veggies include: Increased energy, restful sleep, improved digestion, decreased headaches, hair and nails grow faster and stronger, weight loss and management, more physical activity, lower blood pressure and cholesterol, less aches and pains, lower diabetic sugar levels, and resistance to cancer and disease.

Antioxidants are like microscopic soldiers in your body which defend it from "free radicals". Free radicals are the toxic bad guys that damage our cells and cause disease and aging. There is no better source for antioxidants than fruits and vegetables. These antioxidants attack, neutralize and eliminate free radicals and toxins in the body leading to better health, disease resistance, faster recovery and anti-aging.

Fruits and veggies are living food. They are consumed while they are still "alive". The living enzymes and nutrients in these living fruits and veggies promote life. The living enzymes ingested when we eat raw fruits and vegetables contribute to the "enzyme bank" in our bodies and promote a symbiotic relationship between the enzymes and the host (our body). Our bodies are home to more enzymes, beneficial bacteria and microorganisms than there are people on the planet. Each of these organisms has a specific role they play in our bodies.

Meat is dead when you consume it. As soon as an animal dies, there is a chemical reaction in the animal's body which releases hormones and enzymes that begin the decomposition process. These toxic enzymes remain in the meat and pass into the consumer. It is my belief that consuming dead meat promotes death in the consumer.

What is the difference between a fruit and a vegetable? I classify them based on whether they bear seeds - fruits have seeds and vegetables do not. Examples of fruits include strawberries (which bear their tiny seeds on their skin), tomatoes, avocados, watermelon, oranges, grapes and pomegranates. Vegetables are leaves, beans or roots such as lettuce, spinach, carrots, potatoes, radishes, and peas. Plants and trees bear fruit to perpetuate life. These life giving fruits are filled with seeds that will eventually lead to the growth of other plants which will bear more fruit. When a fruit is separated from a plant or tree, it doesn't kill the plant – it continues to grow to bear more fruit. Leaves give a plant life by absorbing the sun's energy and photosynthesizing it into sugars and food for the plant. Roots give the plant life by absorbing nutrients and water from the soil. It is easy to see how fruits and veggies give life to the plant and that life translates over to the consumer.

In today's mass-market industrialized agriculture, lots of pesticides and fertilizers are used to make plants grow faster and larger. Plants and seeds are even genetically altered and hybrid offspring are formed. These hybrids are often engineered to be seedless or to have other qualities to make them more attractive to the human eye. Although this genetically altered and chemically grown produce may appear more attractive on the surface, what you don't see is all of the chemicals inside. That is why it is especially important to buy locally grown organic produce. In addition to chemical content, this rapidly grown produce often lacks the nutrients and enzymes of their naturally organically grown distant cousins. One reason for this is due to soil depletion. Over-farming of land depletes the nutrients from the soil which are then artificially replaced with petroleum based fertilizers. These fertilizers contain harmful ingredients to the consumer as well as neighboring animals who live in the soil or nearby streams and rivers where rain runoff from the farms pollutes the environment. Do your part to protect your body and the environment – buy only organic products which are grown locally whenever possible.

Juice It

THE BEST WAY TO GET your minimum of 5 daily servings of fruits and veggies is to drink fresh juice. Fresh juice comes directly from fresh fruits and vegetables and is consumed immediately (within minutes of juicing) to get the maximum nutrition. Juicing extracts the majority of the nutrients and enzymes from the fruit or veggie while leaving the pulp out. Basically this translates into an easily digestible drink that is packed full of all of the good stuff your body needs. Drinking your food eases the burden on the digestive system by eliminating all of the solid matter that requires additional digestion and elimination. You go straight to the source and bypass the carrier.

I have been juicing regularly for the last 14 years. Although it is somewhat of a part time job, it has become a habit and part of my daily and weekly routine. I drink mostly several types of juice – wheatgrass, carrot, apple, and tomato. I will occasionally add spinach, celery or ginger to these juices for added nutrition. Juicing requires work – shopping regularly for large quantities of produce, cleaning, cutting and preparing the produce and cleaning and maintaining the juice machine. Juicing is well worth the work involved because the benefits pay high dividends in your health. Drinking a 16 ounce glass of carrot juice is the equivalent of eating about 6 to 8 large carrots. That's a lot of chewing that you don't have to do and a lot of solid waste (pulp) that your body doesn't have to process.

Some personal benefits I can directly attribute to juicing over the last 14 years include:

- My eyesight has naturally improved and I no longer have to wear glasses when I read or work on the computer.

- My seasonal allergies are almost non-existent now.

- My genetic hair loss and receding hair line has slowed down significantly.

- My fingernails grow super strong at incredible speed.

- I have never had a tooth cavity in my life.

- My skin stays healthy and more resistant to sunburn, acne and wrinkles

- I have a high energy level, but operate on less sleep.

- My focus, concentration and motivation get higher every year.

- I get sick less often, and when I do, I recover in a day or so when friends stay sick with the same illness for days or weeks.

These benefits began to become evident within the first year or two of implementing juicing and a vegetarian diet. They continue to improve or maintain the same level due to the cumulative effects of ingesting these vital nutrients daily for a long period of time.

If you have a juicer, here is a great juice recipe to try. It is called **CABALA** juice. It stands for carrot, apple, beet, apple, lemon, apple. Juice 5 pounds of carrots, 2 red apples, 2 green apples, 2 yellow apples, 2 entire lemons, 2 small to medium sized beets. The yield depends on the juice content of the fruit. The shelf life depends on the type of juicer you are using - some may last 24 to 36 hours before losing its potency. But as a rule of thumb, the juice should be consumed immediately to get its full nutritional value.

Juicing is a tough commitment for some people. If you are fortunate enough to live in a community that has a juice bar or health food store that juices, then you are in luck. I get my wheatgrass juice from the local smoothie shop every morning because it is cheaper and easier than buying the grass and juicing it at home. I also enjoy the social interaction and supporting a local business. I juice the rest of my fruits and veggies at home.

If you don't live near a juice bar and do not have time in your busy schedule to shop, prep and clean to get your fresh juice, but want to get the health benefits of fresh juice - then the next chapter will be of great interest to you…

Supplementation

Wᴇ ʟɪᴠᴇ ɪɴ ᴀ ᴡᴏʀʟᴅ full of technology and knowledge that took generations of societies to experience and compile. However, we live in a world that has been pillaged, plundered and robbed of its nutritional value and natural resources.

Our soil has been polluted with pesticides, herbicides and other pollutants. The nutrients in the soil have been depleted due to over-farming and imbalanced farming as well as waste-water runoff.

It is estimated that we would have to eat 28 "organic" apples today to get the same nutrition in just one apple that our grandparents ate 60 years ago. Eating 28 apples requires a lot of shopping and chewing – so what do we do?

The good news is that, although technology has robbed us of "natural value", it has replaced it with some good alternative supplements. I am a huge proponent of natural, raw, organic foods straight from the source - and conversely I am an opponent of ingesting man-made products. But, in certain cases man has done a great job harvesting the best of nature and making it attainable, affordable and convenient without ruining it.

There are some great healthy products available to help supplement our diets with the nutrition that our food may be lacking.

Check out the "Healthy Business" section of the Health and Happiness site on SeanDon.com and discover some healthy companies and their products such as:

- Chews-4-Health

- The Wholefood Farmacy

- Juice Plus

These supplements can give you some of the same nutrition found in fresh juice and raw, organic fruits and vegetables but in a convenient and affordable package.

Grass is Greener

SINCE I AM A VEGETARIAN, people often ask me where I get my protein. My response is to ask them where they get theirs. Most people will proudly reply that they get their protein from eating beef. I then stump them by asking them where the cow gets its protein. The answer is grass. That's right – cows are vegetarian and weigh an average of around 1400 lbs – that's a lot of protein and it is all built by eating grass. So my answer to them is that I get my protein straight from the source – I drink 4 ounces of freshly juiced wheat grass every day. Not only is it a complete protein, but it contains all necessary amino acids that the human body needs. One ounce of wheat grass is estimated to have the same vitamin and mineral content of 2-1/2 pounds of leafy green vegetables. When comparing "apples to apples" and wheatgrass to other fruits and veggies, ounce for ounce it has more vitamin C than oranges and more vitamin A than carrots. Wheat grass is also packed full of minerals such as: calcium, potassium, iron and magnesium. So not only can you spare eating the cow for protein, but can also pass on the milk for calcium too and get both in one shot of grass juice.

Wheat grass is composed of over 70% chlorophyll which carries oxygen to the blood. This oxygen rich blood cleanses, heals and promotes a healthy, disease free environment in the body. Studies have shown cancer immunity in oxygen rich environments. Wheat grass is believed to be one of the strongest anti-oxidants known to man and can rapidly detoxify the body, particularly the liver. This translates into a great hangover cure as well. The increased oxygen content in the blood also promotes physical endurance and stamina.

I have been drinking 4 ounces of wheat grass a day for over 10 years. I can honestly say that it is not the best tasting thing in the world, but my body craves it and has developed a healthy addiction to it. In fact, when I walk into the health food store and smell it being juiced, my mouth starts to water uncontrollably in preparation for what is about to come. Even though it really doesn't taste great, it is a good idea to swirl the wheat grass shot around in your mouth to mix it with the saliva. This begins the digestive process in the mouth and reduces the shock of such a strong antioxidant to the stomach. Wheat grass also contains vital living enzymes which help the body with its metabolism and digestion.

Wheatgrass references date back to the bible in the book of Daniel in which Babylonian King Nebuchadnezzar is cured from illness and insanity by grazing on grass in the same field as the cows did.

Some say the grass is always greener on the other side – I say the grass is greener on the inside. So drink it up!

Recipe for Cancer

THE PURPOSE OF THIS HEALTH guide is to give you information to help prevent cancer, but I will also tell you some sure ways to get it. If you are interested in cooking up some cancer in your body, here is an interesting recipe to follow:

Start by preheating the body to 98.6. Slowly dehydrate over time with a lack of water. Add 12 ounces of syrup, sugar and carbonation (soft drinks). Add just a few dashes at a time of disodium phosphate, potassium sorbate and sodium benzoate (preservatives). Inhale a few free radicals from smoking or second hand smoke or just plain air pollution. Color the concoction with Yellow #5, Red #40 and why not some Blue #1 too. Rinse the body in chlorinated, fluoridated, chemically treated municipal tap water. Seal the mixture in with aluminum zirconium tetrachlorohydrex in a base of cyclopentasiloxane and di-methicone (or just use your deodorant). Do not mix, do not stir and definitely don't run, walk or jump - Let it all sit and stagnate indefinitely. For added protection from sun-spoilage, apply Eicosene copolymer, ethyhexyl palmitate, Octinoxate and some other stuff we can't pronounce (in suntan lotion) directly to your skin and then bake to a golden brown.

If you can't buy these ingredients individually – it's no surprise, because most of them are toxic – but according to government regulatory agencies are "OK" in small quantities when mixed with other stuff. They are readily available at almost any grocer, drug store or convenience store in the form of deodorant, suntan lotion, toothpaste, canned and boxed foods – all for a low and convenient price.

Wake up and smell the roses. You wouldn't put junk or impure gas in the tank of your car – why put junk in your body!?

Cancer's Cure

THE CURE FOR CANCER IS not to get it. In order not to get it, you must understand what causes it. The root of the disease is much deeper than just not smoking or sunbathing. "Cancer" is inherent in nature. We all have it in our bodies right now. The difference between a "healthy person" and a "cancer patient" is that the healthy person's immune system is able to recognize cancer cells and attack and eliminate them while they are in the single-cell stage before they multiply to form new cancer cells thus causing a clump of cancer cells which become tumors.

You could say that cancer is an immune deficiency problem. What causes an immune deficiency in the body so that it cannot defend itself against cancer? I believe it to be overwhelming battles on multiple fronts. The body just gets overwhelmed. I also think lack of "ammunition" such as nutrient rich foods that contain anti-oxidants which assist the body in neutralizing "free radicals" or pollutants contributes to the dilemma. These pollutants in the body can be inhaled in the air we breathe, ingested in the food and water we eat and drink, absorbed through our skin and even produced within our own bodies. That's right – our own body can produce cancer-causing waste through its own metabolic process.

The billions and billions of cells in our body are constantly multiplying through complex DNA chemical chain reactions. One strand of DNA in a cell can contain thousands of chemical sequences that must be perfectly replicated. If one replication goes wrong, the newly formed cell will not be normal and could be deemed cancerous. A healthy immune system is on guard at all times and recognizes the defective cell and eliminates it before it reproduces itself. An unhealthy immune system is deprived of proper nutrients and subjected to pollutants in a body that cannot efficiently cleanse itself of waste. The unhealthy immune system cannot even see the defective cell amidst all of the junk in the body, moreover it is not strong enough to kill and eliminate the cancer cell. Then the cancer cycle begins as the mutant cells then replicate to form more cancer cells and ultimately tumors.

What do you do? Keep your body clean and toxin free on the inside! Drink pure, fresh water by the gallon. Eat tons of fresh, organic fruits and veggies. Avoid known pollutants such as smoke, drugs, artificial food colorings and preservatives as well as chlorinated water. Try to use all-natural and organic products whenever possible. Check out your local health food store and peruse their selection of natural soaps, deodorants, lotions, toothpaste and make-up. Also check out the article on the Whole Food Farmacy on SeanDon.com and browse their web site for all natural products - www.sean.wholefoodfarmacy.com. Keep reading this book!

Remember to tread lightly when discussing cancer prevention and its "non-traditional natural cures" with doctors, nurses, pharmacists, radiologists, chemo therapists and oncologists – they have a lot to lose if cancer is cured. Imagine the economic ramifications on the medical industry if cancer ceased to exist. Trillions of dollars in medical treatments would be unnecessary.

Warning Signs

WHEN YOUR BODY IS UNDER stress from something or a body part is just not right, it sends off warning signs - much like a car's engine knocking when a cylinder or plug is bad. Think about heart burn or indigestion. Your throat (the front door to your body) is burning for some reason and your stomach is upset. Maybe the stomach and throat realize that something does not belong in your body. The brain develops an "allergy" to that substance – whatever it is. This "brain allergy" translates into a burning and churning upper digestive tract. The stomach and esophagus are screaming at you – quit putting (whatever) you are putting into your body. Why would the average person not listen to this?

Think about EVERYTHING you put into your body. Right down to the last hexametaphosphate, monosodium glutamate and yellow #5 (listed on the label of a cheese dip). What the heck are "natural flavors" anyway? How do you make a "natural flavor"? If it is natural and it tastes like blueberry – then why not just list blueberry on the label? Is it possible that there could be just one out of the hundreds of chemicals that the FDA allows to be listed as "natural flavors" and "spices" and "artificial colors" that may be messing up a DNA chain involved in the production and reproduction of stomach and intestinal cells that produce mucus, acid and bile or whatever? What if continued introduction of this "something" into the body will lead to cancer and death – somewhere in the body.

On the other hand, instead of putting the wrong things in your body, maybe you're not giving your body's cells the right ingredients to make and do what it is they are supposed to do. A man can dig a hole with his hands, but give him the right tool such as a shovel and it's much easier and less stressful on him. This same principal holds true with the body. The body needs certain "tools" or ingredients it must get from outside sources such as food, water, air and sunlight. If any of these ingredients are compromised or not given correctly with the right dosage and intensity the body may not function properly. Your body may still "dig the hole with its hands" and barely get the job done, but sooner or later the hands are going to give out. It takes much more to break a shovel!

Why are there so many anti-acid, heartburn and "pink-stuff" ads? Why cover up the problem's symptoms and trade them out for different side effects. I think "side effects" of medicines are the body's emergency broadcast signals changing tone. Somewhere in the back of your brain's recesses is a brain cell saying "Captain, it's unbelievable – we tried to stop the junk intake with heartburn and indigestion, but the stomach and throat now have a thick-slick-pink coat that our warnings cannot penetrate. We have a code three infiltration of the pink stuff! Shall we change course and "allergize" something different, sir?" A microphone cracks and with militaristic authority the order comes to send all available forces directly to the temporal lobes. "Yeah, we'll give us a migraine! That'll teach him to quit putting those things in (this) body! A straight blow to the head – he'll get the message. Begin capillary constriction – now. Good call, captain." So to combat your throbbing head, you throw a few ibuprofen down the hatch and into the bad batch. Next thing you know, it's an all out attack on something else – maybe the liver, kidneys or reproductive organs are next. Are you a listener or a screamer?

If your car's engine started knocking would it be a good idea to try to just quiet it down with a bigger muffler – or maybe wrap the engine in a big pink blanket? A smart driver listens to his car and the warning signs. A small noise or vibration can turn into a major problem if not fixed early on. Imagine eating a hot dog and getting indigestion. Now imagine driving down the highway thinking about your day – almost at your exit – quick glance in the side view mirror, turn signal on, and veering right… Then a horn blasts and you swerve back into your original lane. That other driver gave you a warning sign that saved your (and possibly his) life. Your heart races and you thank your lucky stars that they were watching out when you weren't. That is why horns are mandatory on cars in most states. When used properly a horn is a wonderful communication tool, but don't be the fool who blares the horn in traffic for no good reason!

Could it be that taking pharmaceuticals is like clipping the wires to your body's horn?

If everything and "every-body" were doing their thing correctly and being cool... would there ever be any need for horn blowing in the body or in traffic? If everyone was their perfect weight, just had sex, was exactly where they wanted to be, had ideal surroundings and people they wanted to be with and a healthy meal in front of them... Would there be anyone "honking"? But if there is – Bose just made a wonderful earphone that transmits sound waves to cancel out the outside world. Just don't use them when driving!

The body is full of warning signs and natural defenses. Here are some natural body responses to disease and toxicity.

A fever is the body's defense mechanism for fighting disease and infection. The body is trying to sweat out toxins and put stress on bacteria with heat. Give your body plenty of clean water, fresh air and let it sweat.

Nausea is your body shutting down the digestive system to conserve energy to fight off infection. Or nausea and subsequent vomiting or diarrhea is your digestive system eliminating things that should not be in the body. Go ahead and throw up and get it out of your system. Have you ever felt sick as a dog and then you puke and feel fine?

Coughing is your body trying to get something out of your lungs or throat. Don't suppress it with medicine – encourage it. Hack up that mucus oyster and make room for oxygen to get in.

Diarrhea is a pretty obvious sign that something needs to get out of your intestines. Let it out quickly. Assess what you ate and don't eat it again. Ongoing diarrhea can also mean that your intestines are impacted and coated with something that is not allowing the colon to absorb water from your stool. Do a detox and flood the body with water. If you are having constant diarrhea, your body will become dehydrated rapidly. You need to replace the water you are losing.

A headache usually means the body is dehydrated and the brain is not getting enough blood or O2. You don't get a headache because of lack of aspirin in your body. Stop and listen and fix it naturally – drink water, practice yoga, breathing, inversion and stretching.

Think about this before you fill your next prescription - Antibiotics kill beneficial bacteria too. Your body is home to billions and billions of good bacteria that aid in digestion and other bodily functions. Antibiotics can wipe out colonies of these good bacteria that can take months of good health to replace. This is why it is common for a woman to get a yeast infection after taking antibiotics. The bacteria in her reproductive system that usually attack and eat the yeast are now gone and the yeast take over the joint! Then she has to take more drugs to kill the yeast which will invariably have a side effect on another thing in the body – and so the vicious circle rolls on.

Building Blocks

I LIKE ANALOGIES BECAUSE THEY ALLOW us to think things through logically when they are approached from a different view point. That is why I am going to compare eating food to building a house.

Imagine you are a building contractor and I have just hired you to build a house. Better yet, let's say the house is already built and it just needs maintenance and renovation. There are no complicated plans to read or foundations to dig. The hard part is done… Everything is already built. The house just has some squeaks and creaks and a few leaks. Much like your body could have some strains, sprains, bruises, cancers, arthritis or poor vision. Let's say you have to repair a leaking roof. What materials would you need? It depends on the type of roof, but overall you may need some flashing, caulk, shingles, tar paper, coatings etc… Now let's imagine that the only material available to you is concrete. Besides being extremely heavy, concrete is also porous and absorbs water – making it a poor choice for a roofing material. You could keep pouring concrete on the roof until the weight collapses the structure – or find a new material to properly fix the problem.

Your body is much more complex than any building on earth and needs a wide variety of materials to keep it operating properly. The problem is that most of us are not operating properly, but don't realize it until damage has been done. If your body needs roofing materials (salad) and all you give it to work with is concrete (fast food), then repairs and maintenance cannot be carried out. Your body just stockpiles the concrete (maybe around the waist or hips). Not only does your body not get what it needs, but it gets an excess of what it doesn't need. When materials are obviously stockpiling in the body and other problems still persist, take it as your body warning you that you need to put something else in it!

My second analogy is a termite infested wall (or cancer ridden cells that must be repaired). The wall is made out of wood and is badly deteriorated. We need new wood and nails to rebuild it. Let's compare the new wood to fresh, raw fruits and vegetables and the nails to fresh spring water. Then let's burn the new wood (much like what cooking does to the nutrients in fruits and veggies) and then rust the nails (much like carbonating the water and adding sugar). How strong will our new wall be when made of burnt wood and rusted nails? How many nutrients are we cooking out of our food? How polluted, carbonated, colored and artificially flavored is your water?

Your kidneys and liver are like an air filter in you homes' heating and A/C system. If you don't regularly change the filter, it becomes clogged and the system has to work harder to force air through the dirt, thus increasing your electric bill. If the filter becomes too clogged, it may not let any air pass and may burn up the motor and system. You can't naturally change your body parts, but you can keep them clean and hydrated and assist them with sweat, activity and stretching.

Give your body the materials it needs and it can rebuild itself and keep itself well maintained. Keep it cleansed and detoxified and it will operate more efficiently and stress-free.

Pay to Play

IF YOU ARE GOING TO do things that punish your body such as heavy exertion, smoking, drinking alcohol, sleep deprivation, or stressful lifestyle – then give your body equal or greater rewards to counteract the ill effects.

I like to drink alcohol occasionally, so I made it a habit of drinking at least a 2 ounce shot of wheatgrass juice daily. Wheatgrass juice is a strong antioxidant and can rapidly cleanse and detoxify the liver (which takes a beating from the alcohol).

I also drink copious amounts of mineral rich water to make sure the antioxidants, vitamins and minerals can flow to all of my body and that lactic acid, toxins and waste can be quickly flushed out and eliminated from my body.

I physically work out hard and lead a very active lifestyle with minimal sleep. Therefore, I make sure that I stretch my body out on a daily basis. I even invested in a hot tub to aid in this exercise. Stretching in the morning and night helps to get the blood flowing to muscles and organs. The blood brings in oxygen and nutrients and takes out lactic acid and toxins. My high water consumption also keeps my muscles limber. I find that even though I don't sleep for long periods, I go to bed relaxed and prepared for sleep and wake up feeling energized and loose.

My body's favorite treat is massage therapy. This multiplies the effects of stretching tenfold by forcing blood into tightly knotted muscles. Massage also gets toxins and waste moving from stagnant internal areas in the body. Massage is complimented well with water, stretching, exercise, sleep and fresh air.

Meditation is another form of positive rest and relaxation. Everyone should have a "happy place" where the mind and its emotions can vacation at any time. Those of you who think this idea is juvenile are probably the ones who need it most. Imagine a happy moment in your past – one that you can recall vividly. Where were you? Who were you with? What was the temperature? What smells, sounds, sights, feelings and sensations were around you? Can you imagine this time and place so vividly that the thought actually invokes the same feelings that you felt at that time?

Smiling is another therapy I highly recommend. Try to put on your biggest and most genuine smile and hold it for a minute. Did it change your mindset? It's hard smile when you are in a bad mood, but it is even harder to be in a bad mood when you are walking around with a smile on your face. Scientific research purports that the very act of smiling causes chemical reactions in the body and the release of certain hormones and endorphins. A smile could be a great anti-depressant medicine without all the side effects. Smiling is contagious too. When someone sees you smile, they are likely to do the same in return. Make someone else's day and pass a smile their way.

A day spent upset is a day you might regret. You only have one life to live - better make it positive. So turn that frown upside down and smile for a while!

Skin is a Sponge

Don't PUT ANYTHING ON YOUR skin that you wouldn't put in your mouth. I laugh when I read labels that warn "topical use only" on a medicine or lotion. Don't they know that it is going to be absorbed into your body? The skin is the largest organ in the body and it is also obviously the most visible organ as well. Skin has these little holes in it called pores. The purpose of pores is to let things in and out of the body. Think about what is meant to go in your body through the skin. My answer is… water – pure, clean water.

I believe that sun exposure in limited amounts is healthy and can promote hormone activity and vitamin D production in the body. My rule of thumb is two hours of sun a day – when your shadow is taller than you are (morning and afternoon). Excessive sun exposure at peak times can cause cell damage in the skin and underlying cells. But what if applying sun tan lotion to block out the harmful effects of the sun actually has other less healthy side effects? How many ingredients on your suntan lotion can you pronounce? Do these ingredients occur naturally in nature and do they belong in your body? Who tests these products and their ingredients and do they have any monetary interest in your use of the very product that they test?

Your skin is an excellent tell-tale of your body's health. If your skin (the largest organ in the body) looks unhealthy, chances are that there are "underlying" problems too in the rest of the body's organs. In the past, when you went to the doctor with an ailment (other than trauma) the first thing the doctor would do is tell you to stick out your tongue. He would then examine your tongue and throat. Know what he was initially looking for? The color of your tongue, the presence of plaque and also the smell of your breath is another indicator of toxins (and garlic) in the body.

A healthy, toxin-free body should not emit offensive odors. Sweat, breath, urine and gastric emissions should be free of pungent odor. Fast for several days with water only or fresh juice diet. Exercise, sweat, stretch, sleep while flushing your body with ample water and see what happens to your body odors over the period of several days.

I read an interesting article online a while ago about a study done on people who used suntan lotion versus those who didn't. Not surprising was that the people tested who used suntan lotion had lower occurrences of skin cancer. However, the shocker was that the suntan lotion users had exponentially higher rates of every other type of cancer! Proof-positive that the chemicals in the lotion are being absorbed into the body and causing health problems elsewhere. The study went further to test the levels of vitamin D in people with regular sun exposure versus those with minimal sun exposure. The results showed that when the body is regularly exposed to sun it naturally produces vitamin D. Vitamin D is known to fight and prevent cancer in the body. What an interesting concept – sun exposure causes the body to naturally produce a vitamin to fight cancer!

My theory on sun exposure is as follows. We were born into this world naked. Our skin was meant to protect us from the sun. Melanin in the skin tans us and helps to further protect us from damaging ultraviolet rays. Trees provide shade for us when the sun is at its peak and most intense rays. Different ethnicities who grew up in areas with extensive sun exposure such as the equator and areas with few trees such as the desert, were given extra melanin and darker skin to protect them. My theory also involves my idea that the human race has over-domesticated itself and detached itself from nature. We live in houses rather than nature, we work in an office, wear clothes and hats outside and have limited sun exposure year round. We don't benefit from gradually building up tolerance to the sun and developing a "base tan". Then we take our one week vacation and go to the beach or somewhere tropical. We don our bathing suits on our lily-white bodies and then slather them up with chemical infested suntan lotion and yet still sometimes get burned to a crisp when we swim and wash the lotion off. Furthermore, we don't have the benefit of a vitamin D surplus in the body to help fight off other cancers. Dermatologists will cringe as I say this, but I go to a tanning bed for ten minutes almost daily. I believe that tanning regularly builds up my tolerance to the sun and produces melanin and vitamin D in my skin. I used to burn to a crisp every summer even when I used SPF 45 lotion. Now I can honestly say that I have not been sunburned in years since I started going to the tanning bed. My skin feels great and even looks younger!

Heredity

PEOPLE ARE QUICK TO BLAME their parents and relatives for their health woes. They say the gene pool in their family dealt them a bad hand. I think it is true that some people are more prone to having certain health problems based on physical inheritance from the family, but what most people don't think about are the habits that they inherit as well.

A friend of mine had relegated himself to the fact that he would die of a heart attack because all of the males in his family had heart problems. It was when I attended his family picnic that his problem hit me like a ton of bricks. I looked at his plate - on which he had 2 hamburgers loaded with bacon and cheese, French fries and a beer. I then noticed the exact same fare on his father's plate as well as his uncle's and brother's. Then they all had a cigarette together after they finished eating. Is it just a coincidence that they all ate the same thing at the picnic? I doubt it – there was plenty of fruit and salad and water that went untouched by all of the males at the picnic except me. Like father, like son. It is easier to blame the inherited gene pool rather than give up the hamburger, fries, beer and cigarette!

It is true that we may inherit "weak links" in our genetics from our relatives, but it is the exposure to a toxic or stressful lifestyle that ultimately causes these "weak links" to break, thus making health problems evident. Look at it this way - your genes "load the gun", but your lifestyle pulls the trigger.

Heredity is a great excuse to explain unknown reasons for health problems. I say own up to your actions, be your own boss, retrain your mind and body and quit blaming your family for your health woes.

Know the Truth

FOR THOSE OF YOU WHO want to continue to enjoy the things in life that in the back of your mind you know is bad for you, may want to skip this chapter. There are those of you who would like to eat a hot dog and not think about where it came from, or those who want to enjoy a cigarette without reading the surgeon general's warning label on the side of the package. For those of you who truly care what you are putting into your bodies, I challenge you to trace the origins of your food back to their source. This may be impossible or confounded as so many different ingredients, chemicals and additives come from many sources all over the world. If you shop at your local farmer's market or local butcher store and know the farmer and the location of the farm from which your produce came or if you met the steer before it was slaughtered, then I commend you. You are a minority of less than 1% of shoppers in this country.

Remember in the early days of cigarettes? They were promoted as being healthy and were even endorsed by doctors in tobacco ads. If the price were right, would you agree to do a commercial for something you knew was wrong? What if you just didn't know the facts, but were in a position of authority and influence – would you do the commercial? What if everybody else was doing it and you wanted to support the product to fit in or be cool? What if the price was really, really, really good? What is your price and who do you trust?

Don't take my word for it all. If you truly care about your body and its health, I challenge you to do your own research and draw your own conclusions. I just advise you to know and trust your sources of information. You might be overwhelmed and amazed at the amount of information available to you on these topics. All of the information you find will probably contain many different ideas and contradictory findings. Someone once told me that "opinions are like asses – everyone has one, but some peoples' stink"! Know your own ass and be careful whose you smell.

What I don't trust is the omnipotence of the government agencies and their subsidiaries who test the products that we eat. The organizations that test these products are essentially funded by taxes and fees on the very products they test. Who in these organizations decides what amount of fecal matter or insect parts percentages in our food is acceptable? My tolerance level for feces in my food is zero, but in industrialized food production it is acceptable for a certain number of flies or feces to slip into the ointment so-to-speak.

The interpretation of results of test products on laboratory animals amazes me. I recently read an article on research regarding a link between hot dogs and colon cancer – specifically regarding the nitrates and nitrite in the product and its effect on the colon. Test data showed an increased rate of colon cancer in lab animals, but the test data on humans was inconclusive at this time. Aren't humans animals too? Is it safe to say that if something causes cancer in the colon of a lab rat (an animal at the bottom of the food chain designed to scavenge and eat rotten, toxic food waste) that it probably will cause the same or greater damage in a human colon?

My question is who is testing the testing agencies?

The best advice I can give you is to think intelligently about everything you do regarding your body and its health. Understand and listen to your body and give it what it needs, but be in control of your body and give it what it really needs and not what it craves through addictions or habits. Everyone is different and different things work in different quantities and combinations for different people. Do what makes the most sense and gives you the best results that you are looking for.

Love yourself and be good to yourself and your body will reward you with many years of healthy service.

Brainwashed

WITH KNOWLEDGE COMES POWER. THERE is infinite power in our brains that sometimes never gets recognized or used. We are educated to a certain "acceptable" standard with predetermined government criteria and sometimes that's all we learn. Some people never question what they are taught by their teachers, parents, politicians and laws. But if you think about it, almost everything we are taught came into being because someone questioned something. What if Greek Scholars such as Aristotle and Ptolemy had never questioned the Pythagorean belief that the world was flat and the center of the universe? Would explorers have been brave enough to embark on long voyages for fear of falling off of the edge of the world? What if great minds and inventors had not asked what if…Would we have light bulbs, cars, computers and other inventions? Laws were made because someone challenged the system and did something outside of what was acceptable and then laws were created to prevent that behavior. New languages and cultures evolved worldwide because someone said "What if we do things a little different?"

I once heard a powerful quote: "The best way to keep someone enslaved is to constantly remind them that they are free". In other words, your mind will start to believe what it hears, sees and feels – even if those things are manufactured and introduced to fool us.

Who voted in the election that included the bill to pass the income tax and other IRS laws and powers? Think about all the laws that you question – did you get to vote on them or did your parents or grandparents vote them into law – and why? In the state that I live in, premarital and oral sex is still illegal. I would be willing to bet that a large majority of police, judges, lawyers and politicians in Virginia have partaken in oral gratification and sex before marriage - and still continue to do so. If oral sex was on the ballot this November, would it still be illegal in December?

I briefly dated a pharmaceutical sales rep a long time ago. I was much younger then and didn't have the knowledge and life experiences that I have now, but my brief relationship with her impacted my perceptions and beliefs tremendously. She was a very attractive young lady who dressed well and drove a BMW. In addition to her appearance and material possessions, she also possessed a Bachelor's Degree in marketing and sales from a highly esteemed university. All of these attributes coupled with a very nice income from a successful career in drug sales would have easily been enough to impress the average guy. I was more intrigued than impressed by this girl - mostly because of her constant need to communicate and talk about her job. It's great to love your job and be proud of what you do and naturally you would want to share that with someone who you care about. I was genuinely interested in her and her job, so I listened to what she had to say. What amazed me about her job was her ability to brag about all of the doctors she visited. However, she didn't brag about how great the doctor was or how many patients he saw or how many lives her drugs saved – she bragged about all of the samples she gave to them and all of the prescriptions they wrote for her pharmaceuticals which led to promotions and financial success for her. Often she implied that the doctors simply liked to see her because she was young and attractive or because she also liked to play golf – for free with them, compliments of her employer. She went on and on about how she loved to educate them on all of the new drugs on the market. She would tell me about older doctors she would call on who had graduated from medical school before she was born – and certainly long before the introduction of the new drugs she sold. I bit my tongue and listened, but in the back of my mind thought how crazy it was for a young girl just out of college with a four year bachelor's degree in sales to be educating doctors on drugs. I couldn't help but think that she may have more influence on the treatment that a patient receives than the doctor who went to school for over ten years to get his M.D.

Food for thought: What's up with commercials for drugs that show happy people, flowers, dogs, walks on the beach etc... and don't even tell you what the drug is for - only the name of it. "Ask your doctor if ___ is right for you". And then in a low tone of voice a narrator reads a mile long list of possible side effects at lightning speed. If you did what the commercial showed and danced or took a walk on the beach with your wife, kids or dog – you probably wouldn't need the drug after all and you wouldn't have side effects.

What happens when people rock the boat and question authority? Sometimes they become heroes and martyrs. Others never follow through and give up due to challenges and pressure from society. Some are persecuted, ridiculed and ostracized for their beliefs and new ideas. An unpleasant but well documented part of American history was the witch hunts and stake burnings that took place in the 1600 and 1700s. The irony was that the witches (both men and women) who were imprisoned, persecuted and burned at the stake for their beliefs and new ideas were condemned by people who came to this country as immigrants to escape persecution in their European homeland. Another unpleasant irony is that the USA was founded by men who drafted the Declaration of Independence on the premise that "All men are created equal", but most of these men utilized African slave labor. They also didn't treat women with the same respect as their fellow men. These past atrocities are still brainwashed into our society today and discrimination and reverse discrimination still exist. People are still shunned for new ideas that some may consider unrealistic or not congruent with what they have learned or the religion that they practice.

I say – "wash your brain" of this brainwashing. Open your mind and let new ideas flood in. Think for yourself and use your common sense. Question authority, education and the "written law", but not at the expense of life, liberty, the pursuit of happiness and safety. How many of the laws that you abide by or break on a daily basis did you ever have the opportunity to vote on before they were passed into law? How many ridiculous laws are still on the books today even though they may be outdated and not apply to modern day life? Many discriminatory laws were wiped out of the books during the 1950's and 60's. Women and African Americans can vote, ride the same bus, own property and hold the same jobs as a white man. In fact, Hillary Clinton and Barack Obama were competing to be president of the United States just a mere fifty years after women and blacks were given the right to vote! But do we really still need an affirmative action and equal opportunity law? Should a man not be able to get equal consideration for a job based on his merits and not his skin color whether black, white, red – woman or man – gay or straight?

Let me address another point regarding brainwashing. In this age of technology, all kinds of information is available to us on the internet and through the media. It is more readily accessible and easier to read and understand from the comfort of our living rooms on our personal computers than it was a decade ago. Everyone knows about Google – it is a household word now and I believe it has even been added to some dictionaries. But ten years ago would you be able to go online and Google yourself or another topic and have hundreds of thousands of search results appear on the screen right before your eyes in fractions of a second? Wow – it would be mind boggling to try to explain that technology to someone even ten or twenty years ago. What bothers me is how easy it could be to manipulate a whole population with this newfound technology. As broad, unrestricted and free as the world-wide-web appears to be, I can't help but wonder what would happen if someone with enough money, time and power wanted to change people's perspective on a particular topic or person. If you only got your news from one source (the same TV station, radio or newspaper) you may easily agree that your news could be biased based on the stories that your particular source happened to cover and cram into a one hour show or 100 pages of print or a 30 second news clip. You may also agree that your one source may have certain special interests that would bias their coverage and censorship. If you didn't like the coverage from that source, you could easily change it and start reading a different paper or watching a different news channel. But what if one source could bias the news on a much broader spectrum and make it appear as if it came from many collaborating sources. In this day and age, it is mind boggling to try to figure out corporate conglomerations – what corporation owns what company. So many large corporations own stock in so many different things – and not just for monetary reasons! Influence through constant advertising and persuasion brings a great deal of power.

If a friend made you mad, you may be tempted to send out slanderous emails about that person to all of your friends. You may even write something detrimental on their "Facebook" or "My Space" page to try to retaliate. But what if someone knew something about you and threatened to blackmail you – to what lengths would you go to keep your secret safe? What if you had the power to conveniently bend and impose laws on them and enforce the laws as you saw fit in an attempt to imprison and discredit that person? There are only so many hours in a day to retaliate against someone, but what if you had unlimited financial resources and could hire dozens or hundreds of people to help you in your quest to silence or discredit someone? What if I hired you upon completion of this reading and your job with me was to make sure that no one else ever read this book or web page again? What would you do? Would you take the job? How about if the salary was really, really good? If you took the job, how would you proceed? Would you hire a hacker to break into the web server and wipe out this web page? Would you report me to the AMA (American Medical Association) and try to have me shut down for giving health advice without an M.D? Would you take part of your salary and hire hundreds of people to blog and write bad things about me online and set up web sites to contradict and discredit me and then pay search engines lots of money to make sure your information appeared at the top of their lists and pushed mine so deep into the internet that no one would look that deep to find it? My point is that if it is conceivable, then it is probably just as possible. No more unlikely than the very fact that we have such technology now.

Why does the US have the most medicine, but the worst track record for preventable disease among the top 19 industrialized nations in the world? Why is the American health care system and insurance not affordable to over half of the country's population?

Say What?

I THINK IT IS VERY IMPORTANT to constantly educate yourself. Take everything you hear and see with "a grain of salt". Question the unknown and your sources of information. Understand that everyone has their own beliefs and that different things work for different people at different times. Don't persecute someone for their beliefs, rather accept them as different and respect their opinions as much as you want them to accept yours. Follow the Golden Rule and "Do unto others as you would have them do unto you". Wouldn't the world be so peaceful if everyone adopted this philosophy?

Use common sense and do what is right for you. What is right for you? Where do you want to be in life – now and in five, ten, fifty years? Write down a list of the things most important in life to you and then follow it up with a list of goals that will help bring or keep those important things close to your life. Emulate those who have achieved the goals and live the life that you desire. Once you achieve your goals, lead by example and influence someone else to achieve theirs too.

Assurance

Everyone in modern society knows what insurance is. Most of us write checks every month or year to insurance companies for health, automobile, life, fire, business and personal liability insurances. If you ask me, insurance is the largest form of legalized gambling in our society. Insurance companies are gambling on the fact that you will pay your premiums and not file any claims – and if you do file claims, they may try to evade paying them by imposing deductibles, co-pays and exclusions. Don't rely solely on insurance companies to cover you and don't let your insurance policy be relegated to writing a check for a "paper policy". Start your own assurance policies.

I am not telling you to cancel your insurance policies; however, I am advising you to be your own "assurance agent" every day. Look both ways before crossing the street, don't run with scissors in your hand, eat your fruits and veggies, wash behind your ears, think good thoughts and good things will come your way. Pack your own parachute – or know that it is packed with love by someone who knows what they are doing – if not, you don't know what results you will get when you jump and pull the cord. Don't let the media, commercials, fast food, "drive-thru doctor offices", pharmaceutical companies or uneducated people pack your chute and plan your life for you.

Food for thought – imagine the financial ramifications that curing cancer and other terminal illnesses would have on the medical profession in this country. Doctors, nurses, oncology and hospice care, pharmaceutical companies, X-ray techs, chemotherapy clinics, medical suppliers, insurance companies and even funeral homes would certainly suffer financially. Trillions of dollars of medical treatments would be lost and the need for health insurance would diminish significantly.

A recent study (as published on MSN.com) researched preventable disease in 19 industrialized nations world-wide. France came in first place. The United States… 19th! That's right – 19th out of 19. We have the most advanced technologies in the world and a plethora of pharmaceuticals, yet we have the highest incidents of obesity, cancer, heart problems and other preventable diseases. Ironically, France provides health care at practically no charge to its citizens and visitors. What's the problem with the US? The medical profession makes its living when you get sick and subsequently need medicine and long-term ongoing care! Sad but true.

I am absolutely NOT saying not to go to the doctor. I think doctors are an integral part of health maintenance. I am just advising you to choose your doctor, insurance carrier and health care providers wisely. Take the time to review your doctor's credentials. Interview multiple doctors and find the one that is right for you. You would probably interview and shop multiple lawn care companies, car dealers, electronic retailers and child care providers – so do the same with doctors. Shop and compare, but make price one of your last concerns. After all, good service is worth paying a little bit more for - and what better thing to spend money on than your body. Most importantly, never let a health insurance company tell you what doctors you have to use.

Once you find a good doctor, make it a point to go to him at least once a year for a physical exam. A good doctor will want to see you when you are healthy, not just when you are sick. You should be open and honest about all your health issues and don't be afraid to voice your opinion. A good doctor will take the time to listen and respect your views on your own health, but be authoritative enough to tell you when you are doing something wrong.

The best health insurance is the "assurance" you can give yourself by doing everything within your power to take care of your mind and body.

Weight a Minute

OBESITY IS A PROBLEM THAT is out of control in our society today. It can be blamed for health issues both physically and mentally.

The first obvious problem with being overweight is carrying around extra body mass. Carrying around extra body weight puts more stress on joints that were not meant to hold extra weight. Being fat causes your heart to have to work harder to pump blood through more mass. The extra mass creates more pressure on the blood vessels and lymphatic system and does not allow them to flow freely. This causes blood pressure to rise and the lymphatic system to stagnate and become toxic. To worsen the situation, fat holds toxins.

In addition to causing physical health problems, being overweight can cause mental problems as well. Mentally, being fat can make people insecure about themselves. Overweight people tend to be full of excuses about their weight. They may jump from diet to diet, pill to pill or one exercise to another, but often lack the will power to stick with anything long enough to see results; therefore they quit trying. I think being overweight can also keep someone from doing the very things that will help them lose weight in the first place. I once had a friend that was overweight. She constantly talked about what she was going to do to lose weight, but she never followed through. It is a shame that talking doesn't burn a lot of calories because she would have been slim – fast! I bought her a gym membership for her birthday, but she never used it – because, get this – she said she was too overweight and embarrassed to go to the gym! Unbelievable! Her plan was to work out at home until she felt she looked good enough to go to the gym. Needless to say, it never happened.

I think society should put a little more pressure and motivation on people to lose weight. Airlines and movie theaters should charge fat people double. If you are going to take up two seats, then you should pay for two seats. If you have ever flown cross country next to an obese person, then you can sympathize with how I feel.

I was at an amusement park not too long ago. I stood in line for over an hour behind an exceptionally obese man waiting to ride a roller coaster. When it was his turn to board the ride in front of me, it was no surprise that he could not fit into the car's restraint system. Everyone waited as this guy struggled and had to ultimately exit the car without riding. He seemed very humbled and embarrassed as everyone recognized his dilemma. I wonder if that embarrassing waste of his time in line was enough motivation for him to change his life and lose some weight. Not to sound too crude, but if I was him I would have been walking non-stop through the park, burning calories instead of standing motionless in line for a ride that I couldn't possibly have fit into. The guy, being so large, was pretty hard to miss and later that day I saw him sitting at a patio table with a large pepperoni pizza in front of him. No lesson learned! The pizza must have been too tempting and the desire to be healthy, sit comfortably in a car or an airplane or a rollercoaster was not strong enough.

Here are a few rules of thumb that you should live by to maintain a healthy weight:

- Don't eat a quantity larger than the size of your fist (compressed) for each meal

- Eat 6 to 8 healthy meals a day

- Drink lots of water – it will help curb your appetite

- Avoid everything artificial – box food, can food, artificial ingredients – especially sugar-free items with artificial sweeteners.

- Walk as much as possible. Even parking at the back of parking lots can increase your amount of walking substantially over a month long period. Take the stairs instead of elevators.

- Stand up often when possible. Try to stand for 5 minutes every hour at your desk at work. If you watch TV, try to stand during an entire episode of your favorite show instead of sitting on the couch.

- Hang out with, talk to and watch other healthy people and try to learn their habits.

- Join a gym, travel and get out and get active.

- Find a health food supplement that is right for you – visit the Health and Happiness/Healthy business section on SeanDon. com for some great recommendations.

- Complete a raw food-juice-water fast for at least 36 hours.

The purpose of storing fat is like a bank or rainy day fund for your body to burn during times of drought or famine or pregnancy. The worst thing you can do is eat one or two large meals a day. Your body is programmed and realizes that it may be 12 or 24 hours before another meal comes so it stores everything it can to bridge the gap between meals. If you eat large, heavy meals a couple of times a day, your body never goes out of storage mode. If you eat small quantities of easily digested food every couple of hours, the body will speed up its metabolism and cut down on storage since it knows it has replenishment coming again soon.

Many people get very defensive about their weight or the weight of others. I have heard countless excuses such as glandular problems and heredity. My take on the situation is that obesity is a disease that feeds on addiction, laziness and lack of self control. Obesity is caused by a self-perpetuating cycle of eating unhealthy foods that are packed with addictive chemical additives. This unhealthy food has very little nutrients that your body needs for energy. The junk food also robs your body of a lot of energy just to digest and eliminate the junk. This junk accumulates in the intestines and excess "junk calories" are converted to fat due to lack of calorie-burning exercise and activity. The lack of energy rich nutrients and the loss of metabolic energy causes a more lethargic, sedentary or lazy lifestyle. I call it the "couch-potato cycle".

The couch potato cycle is tough to break and takes a great deal of will-power and stick-to-itiveness. In order to lose massive amounts of weight, you need massive and drastic change in your lifestyle. Rarely do people gain 50 pounds overnight, but rather accumulate it over a period of time. If you didn't gain it over night, don't expect to lose it over night. A lot of people will start diets and work outs only to quit shortly thereafter due to lack of immediate results. Then they fall back into the same cycle that got them the extra weight in the first place.

I think that the best way to break the couch potato cycle is through immediate action, definite and absolute commitment and drastic change. Start with a raw food detoxification. Challenge yourself to eat only raw fruits and veggies and drink only water or fresh juice for 14 days. Consume 6 to 8 meals of raw food per day instead of the typical 2 or 3 meals a day. Drink as close to 2 liters per 100 pounds of body weight per day as possible. You will be hungry, irritable and maybe even feel nauseous or sick at first. That is partly the result of withdrawal from a chemical addiction to some of the foods you have been accustomed to eating. It is also a result of the release of toxins stored in fat being released into the body as the fat is burned. This is why it is essential to drink copious amounts of water to flush these released toxins from the body as rapidly as possible. The body is also going through mental and physical stress imposed by a forced change in metabolism. It will pass and results will develop soon – the time frame depends on how deep in the hole you start and how committed you are to the new program. Have faith and stick with it - the body has an amazing ability to adapt to change.

Let me clarify and define raw food for you. Raw food is uncooked and unprocessed fruits, vegetables, nuts and grains. A salad is raw, but cannot contain cheese, egg or salad dressing or anything else other than veggies and fruits. If you must use a salad dressing, use only extra-virgin olive oil and spice up the salad with fresh ground pepper and fresh herbs such as cilantro, basil or dill. Leave out the iceberg lettuce as it has very little nutrients and use green and red leaf lettuce, baby greens, arugula and spinach – hey Popeye was on to something! Ideally, your salad should have a wide variety of veggies and it should look like a colorful rainbow. Raw fruits come in their peel or skin and not a box, can, carton or wrapper. Raw juice comes fresh from the fruit or vegetables. Once the fruit or veggie is juiced, it begins to break down rapidly and lose its potency. When fruits and veggies are cooked, many of the nutrients are altered and lose their effectiveness. So eat them fresh – and eat them often!

As you detoxify, you will find that you will start to have more energy. You wake up feeling more refreshed – maybe even before the alarm clock goes off. You will also become more focused and alert. Your metabolism will naturally speed up. The raw food will be digested easily and will take less energy to process and eliminate. The increased water and roughage intake will begin to shed impacted waste in the intestines – clearing a path for nutrients to be absorbed, thus increasing energy levels. Now the detox cycle has begun. Keep the cycle going and ultimately you will reach your ideal weight.

Once you break the couch potato cycle and start the detox cycle, another interesting phenomenon occurs. In addition to physically feeling better, your mentality changes too. You start to feel a sense of accomplishment and feel proud of yourself. You will find yourself looking in the mirror more to see progress. You will brag about your successes and weight loss to friends, coworkers and family. You will be the one to motivate others to do the same. You will become resistant to temptations and influences from other people.

I have never been overweight so I am speaking from observations and common sense, but I have worked very hard all of my life to maintain my weight. I think there is too much hype and undeserved congratulations for people who get fat and lose a lot of weight. There are even TV shows that turn weight loss into a competition. However, I do like to be a positive influence on people and I am more than happy to share my details that have kept me slim and fit all of my life. Where is the credit and congratulations for the people that stayed healthy and slim and never got fat? The satisfaction should be in the way you feel and look!

Game Plan

ONE OF MY FAVORITE QUOTES comes from Anthony (Tony) Robbins - a very influential person who happens to be a world renowned motivational speaker. In his books and seminars, he reminds us of Albert Einstein's definition of insanity: "to continue doing things the same way, but expect different results." How true! Most of us want to change and want different results in our lives, but either lack the will power and motivation or simply don't know what to do and how to do it. Hopefully you have the will power within and maybe my writings will help motivate you to make positive changes in your life. And just so you don't have any excuses not to change, I have outlined a game plan for you to start with. Remember everyone is different and different things work for different people, so listen to your body and do what feels right and gives you the results you are looking for. My attorney has advised me that I need to have a disclaimer in my writing to protect myself legally. I should tell you to "contact your physician before trying any new natural diets or workout plans to make sure that your body is capable of withstanding the change". I say… "How can a doctor possibly know your body better than you? If you die from following my advice, you were going to die anyway - hopefully you passed away healthier and happier. What doesn't kill you makes you stronger!"

Detoxification: Your first goal and primary focus should be on detoxification of the body. Wipe the slate clean so that you can start over fresh. The emphasis will be on water, fresh juice, light exercise, sweat, stretching, meditation and sleep.

Water: Make it your goal to drink one liter per 50 pounds of body weight daily. A two hundred pound person would need four liters of water a day. I recommend FIJI water which is sold in six-packs of 1 liter bottles. One liter should be consumed first thing in the morning when you wake up and one liter should be consumed at night before sleeping. The rest of your water intake should happen regularly throughout the day. Always keep a bottle of water with you. Never let yourself get thirsty. Set your watch alarm to go off every 30 minutes to remind you to drink. Often our bodies mistake thirst for hunger – drinking ample water will suppress hunger and aid in metabolism while flushing toxins out of the body. You may think that consuming a six pack of FIJI water on a daily basis at an average cost of $2 per liter may be expensive – I challenge you to find a cancer patient and ask them how much time and money their disease has cost them.

Fresh juice: Is not purchased in cartons at the store. It is not canned, cooked, flash-pasteurized, colored, sweetened, filtered or preserved. It comes from fresh organic fruits and vegetables straight through a juice machine and into a glass for your immediate consumption. To get all of the nutritional benefits of juice, it should be consumed immediately as it loses its potency rapidly once removed from its parent source. You may find it inconvenient to have to go to the local juice bar or buy your own produce and juice it yourself and then have to clean the juice machine, but I challenge you to find someone with kidney failure who has to go to a medical facility on a daily or weekly basis to have dialysis done. Ask them about inconvenience.

Light exercise: Exercise is probably the first thing to get bumped on a busy and stressful day. Ironically, it is probably the most important thing in your battle with stress and detoxification. Regardless of your current level of fitness, the goal is to get your body moving on a regular basis. Refer to my Flexercise chapter for exercises that can be done while multi-tasking. This chapter contains simple exercises that can be incorporated into your daily routine with minimal time requirements. A bare minimum of 60 minutes a day should be devoted to some form of exercise. Ideally, split 60 minutes into 3 twenty minute sessions throughout the day. Stretch and flex while in traffic on the way to work. Stand at your desk at work and bounce from heel to toe (rebound exercise). Walk – intentionally park at the back of the parking lot, bike instead of driving if possible, forget about elevators and take the stairs. For those of you who work out rigorously already, good job – keep it up. For those of you who take your legs for granted and don't use them – go visit an amputee or a paraplegic.

Sweat: Depending on your level of physical exertion, this may be satisfied with light exercise. If not, visit a sauna, steam room or hot-tub. Most gyms and neighborhood spas have saunas. It is worth the cost of the gym membership simply to use the sauna. Sauna temperatures may range from 120 degrees to 220 degrees Fahrenheit. I have found my best range to be from 180 to 210. My goal is to stay in the sauna until I feel that I have sweated out ¼ of the water I have consumed that day. Sometimes I feel that my body does this the minute I walk into the sauna, other times I may stay in up to 20 minutes at a time. Important tip: if you feel nauseous, light headed or dizzy exit the sauna immediately and lie on a cool surface with a cool, damp cloth on your forehead. DO NOT lie down in the sauna if you feel tired or dizzy. It may be best to sauna with a friend at first who can monitor you and help you in the event that you should pass out or have adverse reactions. Ironically, from my observations, the people who have adverse reactions to saunas are the ones who need them the most. I consume, on average, one liter of water during a twenty minute sauna session and my goal is to sweat out at least one liter of water during that twenty minute session. How do I know how much I sweat out in the sauna? There is digital scale with one decimal point in the locker room of my gym right outside of the sauna. I weigh myself before I go in and weigh myself as soon as I come out. I then weigh a one liter bottle of water and factor in the minimal weight of the plastic bottle. A gallon of water weighs 8 pounds. There are approx 4 liters of water in a gallon, so therefore each liter of water should weigh about 2 pounds. Theoretically, I should weigh the same when I exit as I did when I entered even though I consumed 2 pounds of water while in the sauna. I weigh 200 pounds, consume at least 4 liters of water daily and sweat out one liter (2 pounds) in twenty minutes. If weight loss is your goal, don't get too excited – this is only water weight and should be immediately replenished. The goal is to sweat and flush toxins, not lose water weight. Weight loss will be inevitable as a result of detoxification. If time is short in your day, try to multi-task and incorporate stretching and meditation into your sauna routine.

Goals: The most vital part of your game plan should be to set some personal goals and write them down. Make your goals specific, realistic and attainable. If necessary, use your goals to invoke massive change in your usual routine and break bad habits. This goal setting should be followed by plans of action. It is one thing to set a goal to walk on your lunch break every day for one hour. However, the reality is that you have to eat lunch and that may outweigh the importance of walking. So, following up your goal with a plan of action such as: I will pack a lunch every morning consisting of healthy items that can be consumed easily during work throughout the day, thus freeing up my lunch hour to be devoted to walking, not eating. I will change my grocery list and include items such as apples, grapes, carrot sticks, granola and bottled water.

Achieving your goals should become your primary focus and everything you do during the day should keep you on your path to success.

Will Power Will Empower

WILL POWER IS PUTTING YOUR mind to something, doing it and sticking to it. The first step is to write a list of small, attainable goals. The next step is to develop a strategy, plan of action or "to-do" list to help you accomplish your goals. The third step and hard part is starting your strategy and eliminating distractions in your life that will keep you from following through with your plans. Prioritize your tasks and devote the most time and effort to the ones that will produce the greatest results. Focus on things within your control and change them to fit into your strategy. When you start to change things within your control, those things previously out of your control may follow suit.

Success and accomplishment will empower you to achieve more and continue positively. Once you experience how good accomplishment feels, it will motivate you to do more. Don't be afraid to take credit and reward yourself if you achieve a goal. However, don't make the reward detrimental to what you are trying to accomplish. For instance, I had a friend that would reward themselves with dessert after dinner – if they went to the gym that day. That reward seemed pretty counterproductive, since their goal and whole reason for going to the gym was to lose weight!

One of the most inspiring things I have ever done was to walk through 40 feet of hot, burning, flaming coals barefooted. This incredible stunt took place at a Tony Robbins "Superself" seminar. Tony teaches you to unlock your mind and use its power to accomplish the impossible. Unbelievably, I walked through those flaming coals at a slow, methodical pace while imagining I was walking on cool, wet sand at the beach. After I accomplished that feat with absolutely no burns or even singed hairs on my feet, I started to question what other impossible things I could accomplish.

It is amazing what the body can accomplish when the mind wants it to.

Sweet Emotion

THE ONLY THING YOU TRULY have control over in your life if your attitude. If you want to make one profound change in your life - focus on what you can control and start with your attitude because it is the only thing you have 100% total control over. Your attitude directly affects your emotions. Your attitude and emotions affect your life. Positive, happy people tend to have far more opportunities come their way than negative people. Think about it – negative people tend to be a drag. Who wants to hang around them? If hearing how miserable someone else's life is makes you feel better, then maybe you need to reevaluate your definition of happiness. Pleasant, positive, happy people attract the same kind of people. Conversation and interaction with positive people leads to positive opportunities and relationships.

In my opinion, there are 3 different kinds of people in the world:

- The first type of people are the ones I want to be forever associated with – they are the people who want to be happy and make those around them happy too. They find personal happiness in the happiness and success of others.

- The second type of people want to be happy too, but are willing to be happy at any cost – even at the expense of other's happiness and well being. These people may even find happiness in the misery and failures of others.

- The third type of people truly want to be miserable. They don't know how to be happy or even what true happiness is. Misery is their comfort zone - and since misery loves company, they want to make everyone around them miserable too.

Be a happy "glass is half full" kind of person and you will find that your glass is constantly getting refilled by others. Do your best to impart happiness on others. Lead by example – your positive energy may rub off on them. If there is a person who you care about and they are "thirsty" and need a drink from your glass from time to time – then by all means, share! Everyone needs some help, motivation and encouragement from time to time, but if there is someone in your life who is constantly drinking all of your glass without ever refilling it, or worse, trying to dump your glass out – then distance yourself from that person. You will be doing both of you a favor. Sometimes the best thing you can do to help someone is to cut them off and let them fend for themselves. As the old saying goes – "You can take the horse to the water, but you can't make them drink". I say – if someone gets thirsty enough, they will find the water themselves and drink until they are fulfilled. Finding the water and drinking by themselves may be the empowerment and self confidence boost they need.

Know that everything you do matters and makes a difference to someone or something. If you don't believe me, watch the DVD "The 7 Decisions" by Andy Andrews. Also, Google the Butterfly Effect and read about this interesting theory.

If you think your life is horrible, if you think you have bad luck, and if you think things can't get any worse – you will be surprised how wrong you are.

If you have lost a loved one, cherish the memories – for they are the most valuable thing that can be inherited from someone. Use their energy that you gained from life with them to carry on their legacy vicariously through yourself. The highest respect and compliment you can pay someone is to imitate or emulate them.

Live and appreciate life every day. There is no such thing as a bad day, only a better one! Learn to control your attitude and emotions and you will be amazed how increased control over other aspects of your life will follow. True wealth is found in the heart and mind, not the pocket, purse or bank.

Flexology

BEING INFLEXIBLE CAN BE NEGATIVE on our bodies in many ways. Being inflexible or unable to adapt to situations can cause us pain and hardship mentally and emotionally. For instance, not being able to get over an ex boyfriend, girlfriend, husband or wife can cause great mental and emotional stress. Life throws curve balls at us and we have to be ready to knock them out of the park with success. Flexibility exudes the ability to change, adapt, assess situations and make the proper move to succeed or get out of harm's way. If you can successfully bend your thoughts, ideas and plans in a slightly different direction, you will go around the obstacle that was blocking your path to success. Those who can't bend or change direction either plow head first and crash into the problem or try to bend and end up snapping.

Physical flexibility can be just as important as mental flexibility. In order for the brain to function at its peak, it must be free from the stress of pain caused by tension. The body is strong, yet sensitive and delicate in many ways. The body has an unbelievable ability to protect and heal itself when it is in total sync with the brain. If the brain gets distracted with mental and emotional pain, it is easy for it to let the body's immune defense system down. Likewise, when the body is constantly screaming pain, the brain will have a hard time dealing with mental and emotional issues. Physical pain derived from injury or stress can cause emotional issues and lead to irritability, depression and even suicide.

When the brain is happy and operating free from stress, it is likely to keep check on the body and keep its systems working properly. The brain is eager to tell the body what to do to stay healthy and protect itself. This kind of brain messaging could cause us to do something drastic... like smile! Smiling leads to adrenaline, endorphin and hormone release in the body. This release gives us energy and "motivation" to go out and do the things that will keep us healthier... such as exercising, making love, smiling more, laughing, being active and burning calories. A happy and flexible person tends to walk more upright and maintain a better posture, thus leading to spinal balance.

How does one become inflexible? Not hydrating the body leads to tight, cramped muscles. Sitting in a chair at a desk, driving a car, slumping on the couch for hours during a movie or video game does not use, much less stretch the body. If you don't use it, you lose it. The muscles begin to tighten which constricts blood flow. The constricted blood flow brings less oxygen to the brain and organs and carries fewer toxins away. Your muscles tighten further and pull your spine out of whack. The misaligned spine pinches nerves that carry vital information from the brain to all parts of the body. All of a sudden the intestines get attacked by a virus or bacteria and the body can't get word to the brain to send in the white blood cells and activate the immune defenses. Next thing you know you are sick... and you have an aching back and headache. Now your aching head makes you grumpy and "short" with your companion. Now you are in an emotional battle which causes more stress and tension in the body. And then you run into some financial woes... which make you work harder and longer and thus spend less or no time at the gym or with the family and friends. You become further removed and detached from what is healthy. Maybe you turn to drinking or smoking to relieve the stress and tension. Then you load your body up with more toxins and carcinogens. When these free radicals are released into the body they tax the body's resources and immune system as it fights to get rid of them or work around them. Next thing you know, these toxins build up and disrupt a cell replication in your body. But the body's immune system can't respond because it doesn't get the massage due to a road block in the spine or it gets stuck in a traffic jam of free radicals as it tries to get to the deformed cell. The white blood cells that were supposed to respond and eliminate the defective cells were tied up fighting with other intruders such as bacteria, viruses, toxins and free radicals. The defective cell is not destroyed and replicates into 2 cells, and they form 2 more and 2 more and so on and so forth... next you develop a tumor. Then that tumor leads to ultimate mental stress - imminent death.

Here is another example of mental inflexibility. You fail to learn new technology at your job and get replaced by someone else who has the skills, or even worse, you get replaced by a computer. Mental stress is activated and the cycle starts over. You can't seem to get a date which causes lack of self confidence and slouched posture which causes added pressure on a lower back that hasn't been stretched or exercised in months or years. The delicate muscle or joint or disk in your back tears and sends pain screaming to the brain... and the cycle continues.

How does one become and stay flexible? Attaining and maintaining flexibility will require some dedication and discipline. If you are ill and in pain, odds are that unless you suffered some form of trauma, you probably didn't get that way from one particular instance or only one source. So, to correct inflexibility it will take more than one cure or practice. I recommend acupuncture as one of them. Acupuncture has the ability to pinpoint imbalances in the body's energy flow. It can also target a particular pressure point that can release energy, tension and stress and send a vital message to the brain that attention is needed somewhere in the body. Some naysayers will tell you that acupuncture is hokus-pokus, but the practice has been an integral part of Eastern medicine for thousands of years. From my personal experience, I can tell you that it works – especially when combined with lots of water, restful sleep, stretching or yoga, chiropractic treatment, exercise and massage. I have walked into an acupuncturist's office with a splitting migraine headache and, after a few hair-like needles were placed in my body without me even knowing it, I emerged from the place pain-free and smiling with a hint of incense lingering in my nose.

If you are past the point of physical injury in your spine, then you may need some assistance from a chiropractor or doctor to get it straight again. Depending on the gravity of your situation, this may take multiple treatments through an ongoing commitment of stretching, hydrating and maintaining a positive posture. It is hard to put out the fire in a raging backache if you keep throwing fuel on it.

Here is my tree branch analogy- The tree and its' branches that stay watered, well fed and nourished will remain flexible and bend in the wind and ultimately grow to become so strong that they cannot be broken except by profound forces of nature. The branches that are dehydrated and deprived of nutrients will snap off in the slightest breeze.

Flexercise

"**F**LEXERCISE" IS A TYPE OF exercise I came up with during times in my life when I was short on time or found myself stuck in traffic or other confined places where traditional exercise was not possible. Flexercise is also a perfect starting workout for couch-potatoes.

Flexercise uses your body's natural resistance from opposing muscles to flex and stretch itself. Clench your fist, bend your arm at a 90 degree angle and flex your bicep while simultaneously trying to pull your arm back straight with your triceps. Create your own resistance with a battle between these two opposing muscles. Then try the same thing with your upper legs in your quads and hamstrings. While sitting upright, bend slightly forward and flex your abdominal muscles – then engage your back muscles and try to slowly pull yourself upright again while maintaining flex in your abs. Lift your arms overhead and engage your shoulder muscles to keep them held high – then slowly try to pull your elbows to your sides with your lat muscles without releasing your shoulders. Flex your calf muscle and point your toe, then engage the muscle in your shin and try to bring your toe back to your shin bone without releasing the calf. Hold the flex as long as you can and breathe deeply as you do it.

Stay loose and stretch your body as often as possible. Plant your feet in one spot, stand tall and release your hips and start to rotate your upper body from side to side. Flex at the waist, alternating sides - then allow your arms to swing side to side with your motion. Allow the weight and centrifugal force of your swinging arms to pull your twist further around each time. Breathe deeply with each twist. Feel the twist loosen your body and your spine. Your internal organs will benefit from the motion as your core muscles engage and force toxins out of the organs. The motion will stimulate the lymphatic system and begin to circulate and move toxins out of the inner body. Imagine your body as a wet towel and the twisting motion is wringing the water out of the towel.

I also highly recommend taking Yoga classes and regularly performing the poses. They are energizing, detoxifying, yet relaxing to the body.

The results of "Flexercising" will be proportionate to your commitment to doing the exercises. No gym, no equipment, no workout clothes, no extra time - no excuses required to incorporate this into your day.

Stress Less

RELAXATION IS NECESSARY TO COUNTERACT the effects of stress on the body. Relaxation has different meanings to different people. Some may consider walking or reading a form of relaxation. Others may watch a sunset, meditate or practice yoga. Sitting on the couch watching TV with a beer in hand may be relaxing to some as well. My definition of relaxation is anything that puts the mind and body at ease and reduces stress. There are positive and negative forms of relaxation. For instance, sitting on the couch with a beer in hand may give you a sensation of mental relaxation, but certainly does nothing physically for the body. Meditation, deep breathing, stretching and yoga relax the mind and body and gets blood and oxygen flowing throughout.

I think it is important to keep stress in check in your life by learning to separate stress from responsibility, obligations, and problems. Change your perception of your life and realize that you have control over your attitude and your attitude is based solely on your PERCEPTION of things. If you constantly perceive your job or responsibilities in life as problematic, then your perception will likely affect your attitude negatively which is sure to trigger stress.

Stress is absolutely the most detrimental thing to your health. In fact, I once heard about a study that was done on four different groups of random people. All of the four groups were initially examined and then tested at the beginning of each daily session for body fluid Ph, hormone levels and toxicity. Group one, the control group, was brought in daily for several hours and just sat in a room at room temperature with normal lighting, normal sounds and no responsibility or tasks to do. Group two, the smokers, were put in the same environment as the control group with the exception being that they smoked cigarettes and were exposed to each other's second hand smoke during their testing time. Group three, the drinkers, drank alcohol instead of smoking. Group four, the stress group, did not get to smoke or drink. Instead, they were placed in a room where the temperature changed dramatically and sporadically, they were subjected to random noises, flashing lights and were asked to solve difficult puzzles and math problems. Would you be surprised to learn that the stress group had more toxicity and higher Ph levels in their bodies than the other three groups combined?

Statistical evidence suggests that when our country enters into an economic recession, health problems increase. I think this is due to two factors. First, the stress caused by financial problems can wreak havoc on the mind and body. And second, people are forced to make sacrifices due to lack of money. Usually one of the top sacrifices is the quality of food which we purchase. The dollar menu at a fast food restaurant becomes the best option instead of healthy, fresh organic foods. Trying to save money by eating cheap food will usually result in greater expense later in medical bills or reduced income from time lost at work due to illness.

Stressful times are the very times when we need to be most diligent in our efforts to maintain health and combat the effects of stress. If we let stress take control of our bodies, we will lose our health and cause a much higher level of stress. Exercising, eating nutritious foods, drinking plenty of mineral rich water, smiling, stretching, yoga, meditation, walking, talking to loved ones and restful sleep are some ways to fight stress.

My favorite way to relax is vacationing. Everybody loves a vacation – the very word brings thoughts of happiness, rest and relaxation. My favorite way to vacation is to take a cruise. I like cruising because just about every major cruise line outfits all of their cruise ships with spas and gyms. In the spa you will find all kinds of options for detoxification – from mud baths to steam rooms, saunas, massages, reflexology and facials – relax and be pampered! In the gym you will find free weights and nautilus equipment as well as treadmills and stationary bikes. Some cruise ship gyms even have boxing rings and punching bags for those you really need to knock out some pent up stress. The cruise ship gym usually offers a variety of classes including yoga, Pilates, and aerobics. If a gym doesn't appeal to you, how about walking on deck and breathing in fresh sea air – or just lying out by the pool resting and soaking up the sun's vitamin D producing rays?

Contact your travel agent and plan your next stress relieving vacation now. If you don't have a travel agent, I recommend Cruise Escapes by Beverly Bell. Check out the following link to Cruise Escape's web site. You can book your way into relaxation on line at www.cruiseescapesbybeverlybell. com

Get out there and explore the world and enjoy life. Make some new friends, see some new places and cultures and give your mind a break from the stresses of your daily routine.

Have you ever been stressed out while on vacation? – I didn't think so!

Heart Health

THE HEART IS A MUSCLE and if you don't use it, you lose it. This muscle beats, on average, 4200 beats per hour, 100,800 beats per day, 7 days per week, 365 days a year - constantly. It never gets a break because if it did, we would die. This ultra-important muscle is the symbol of love, but often is neglected love itself. We need to take care of the muscle that makes us tick.

The irony is the heart symbol not only portrays love, but is also the target of heartache from loss of love. The heart can suffer greatly from emotional stress which can cause a myriad of health problems including, heart attack, hypertension, high blood pressure and more. Compound the effects of stress on the heart by adding alcohol and smoking to cope with the stress - along with an unhealthy diet and maybe a hereditary predisposition for heart problems and you have a recipe for disaster.

Almost 3000 people die from heart related problems daily - that's a football stadium full of people every month and over 650,000 people per year making heart disease the biggest killer in the USA - accounting for over 27 percent of all deaths in our country. Most of these deaths were the first symptom of heart attack or the first sign that there was any problem in the first place. Heart disease is the silent killer and often gives no warning signs or second chances.

More and more young people are dropping dead from heart attacks - the first time. This could be due to the fact that their bodies have not had time to properly adjust to sudden changes in stress levels or the influx of toxins or pollutants that quickly harden and clog blood vessels. Young people are more likely to be killed by the initial heart attack now than some elderly people because their bodies have not had time to slowly adapt to hardening and clogging arteries gradually over time and build alternate pathways for blood to continue to flow past blockages.

Many doctors will prescribe a daily dose of aspirin to help prevent heart attacks, but aspirin has side effects including ulcers and kidney damage. There is an alternative to aspirin. Nobel prize winning research shows that L-Arginine, an amino acid, can possibly help prevent heart attack by keeping arteries flexible and dilated while preventing blood from clotting in the arteries. Arginine is essential to our diet and required for life and has no known toxicity. It has been shown to stimulate the body's production of Human Growth Hormone (HGH) by the pituitary gland which can block the secretion of HGH inhibitor somatostatin. Studies have shown that oral arginine boosts immunity, fights cancer, promotes healing, protects and detoxifies the liver, improves thymus function, and enhances male fertility. Arginine is also used by the body to heal wounds, help the kidneys remove waste from the body and maintain immune and hormone function. Should you decide, in consultation with your physician, to replace your daily aspirin with 3-6 grams of oral arginine, you may notice some other interesting effects as well. One effect in particular may negate the need for men to spend upwards of $10 on a Viagra pill. Some foods that naturally contain this amino acid include nuts (hazelnuts, walnuts, pecans, Brazil, cashews, peanuts, almonds), seeds (sesame, sunflower), brown rice, coconut, raisins, and grains (barley, buckwheat, oats, corn). Visit the "healthy business" section of Seandon.com for other supplements containing arginine.

Aside from supplementation of arginine, there are other profound things you can do to keep your heart healthy. Keep your stress to a minimum and get plenty of restful sleep. Avoid greasy, fatty fried foods and fast food. Use only the purest 24 karat salt (as explained in the Salt's Fault chapter). Don't drink acidic, caffeinated beverages such as sodas and coffee. Flex your heart muscle daily and exercise to elevate your heart rate for a bare minimum of twenty minutes daily. Visit your doctor regularly for checkups and monitor your blood pressure and cholesterol level. Breathe deeply and maintain good posture to allow your lungs to fully oxygenate the blood. Stay flexible and hydrated. Find passion in something productive in your life.

Give your heart the love that it deserves and it will return the favor with billions of life-giving beats.

The Amazing Programmable Body

IT IS AMAZING HOW ADAPTIVE the human body can be. It can also be strong and resilient with the right ingredients. One of the most important ingredients is mental health.

A positive attitude can lead to positive habits which can lead to positive health.

The body can be equally negatively influenced by stress and bad habits. Stress is the single most detrimental element to the body.

It is relatively easy to form a habit both good and bad. It takes mind over body control to determine which habits are beneficial and which ones are detrimental. It takes a great deal of will power to overcome temptation and addiction. The power to change is physically possible if it is backed by mental strength and awareness. The body has the ability to heal both physical injury and overcome terminal illness. The mind has the ability to direct the body to heal itself. Sometimes the hardest thing to heal is the mind because the mind can't see its own faults. Sometimes the mind's own faults cause it to not recognize physical distress. Mental and emotional pain can be more detrimental than trauma or disease in that it can cause the body's natural defense system to be compromised and weak.

The body becomes programmed to accept what it is accustomed to. Your eating habits program your metabolism. If you feed your body three meals a day at the same times with a specific quantity of food, then your brain and digestive system come to expect that and plan accordingly. However, your metabolism dictates your body's ability to process and eliminate food. If your mind makes the decision to reprogram the body, the body may object, but if the mind remains steadfast, the body will adapt.

The most strenuous activity your body is exposed to sets the tone for your endurance and strength. If your most strenuous activity is getting off of the couch to go to the fridge or bathroom, then anything more demanding than that becomes stressful and difficult and can tire you easily. If you climb mountains for exercise, then anything less than that becomes easy.

Learn to reprogram your body as if it were as easy as changing channels on TV. Remember that the definition of insanity according to Einstein is "to continue doing things the same way, but expect different results." Let your mind empower your body and let your will power reinforce your decisions to make changes and stick to them.

Moderation

IF YOU BREAK THE WORD moderation down you get "mode" and "ration". To me, the word means to be in the mode to ration – or have the state of mind to limit quantity.

If you must drink alcohol, ration yourself and drink to a point of enjoyment but stop short of detriment (or excessive drunkenness). You will find that rational drinking will be a lot more enjoyable than excessive drunkenness. Not only will you prevent damage to your health and avoid hangovers and morning sickness, but others may also find you to be a more pleasant person to be around.

If you must eat candy or junk food, moderate it. The same applies to smoking or other unhealthy habits. However, be advised that once the toxins in these substances enter the body they can stay there for long periods of time (some for 15 years) before they can be naturally processed and eliminated from the body. Moderation does not help the cumulative effect of toxic build up in the body. If you only smoke one cigarette a day, there are still 365 days in a year and at the end of the year you have the toxins of 365 cigarettes in your body. It only takes one toxin in the wrong place at the wrong time to cause a health problem.

Eating healthy and exercising and following other healthy suggestions in my writing can help speed up the detox process, but letting these toxins into your body even in small quantities can still do big damage.

If you have to stop and ask yourself if what you are doing is right or wrong, the answer is probably evident just by asking the question in the first place.

Salt's Fault

SALT IS ESSENTIAL IN YOUR body's health and maintenance. Made up of sodium chloride (NACL), it provides the ingredients for necessary chemical reactions in the body. For instance, stomach acid is hydrochloric acid (HCL). Chloride from salt is used to make this acid. Salt also helps the body to retain its water. Salt is also the best know natural astringent and anti-biotic. After you have dental work done, such as a tooth removed, the dentist may tell you to gargle warm salt water. Gargling warm salt water can also cure a sore throat. Have you ever cut yourself or had a skin blemish that healed rapidly after swimming in the ocean?

The fault of the typical mass-produced granular table salt is in the mining and refinement process (or lack thereof). Modern day, mass-produced salt is strip mined from quarries. During the mining process, the salt is excavated along with other things such as rock particles and quartz. The white granules of salt we buy at the store and use in our cooking have many impurities in them. If you were to look at salt under a microscope it would appear to have shards of glass and metals in it. These microscopic particles along with the salt are absorbed into our bodies. The tiny shards get into our blood vessels and tumble along - cutting the walls of the blood vessels. These internal cuts cause two problems. First, the tiny cuts cause scar tissue to form through the body's natural healing process. Second, our body triggers a natural defense mechanism by forming its own cholesterol to patch the scar tissue and line the blood vessels to stop the damage from occurring. The cholesterol lining coupled with the scar tissue causes the areas inside the blood vessels to shrink and even become blocked, thus raising our blood pressure. The heart has to work harder to pump the blood and less oxygen laden blood gets to where it needs to go.

If you cut salt out of your diet to stop this process, then you take away a vital element in your diet leaving your body without the ingredients it needs to carry out its natural chemical reactions. Furthermore, you also take away a natural anti-biotic which leaves you more susceptible to infection. So what's the solution to this dilemma?

In ancient times, salt was graded like gold. The refinement process of salt was much more thorough and deliberate in past history. It was mixed with pure water and strained through cloths and dried in the sun to remove impurities. Have you ever heard the saying "I earned my salt today?" That came from ancient times when people were actually paid wages in salt. Salt was important in past civilizations before refrigeration was conceived. It was used to cure meats and foods and preserve them naturally for later consumption.

I use a raw, pure, "24 karat" salt that I purchase from a natural foods company called the Wholefood Farmacy (www.sean.wholefoodfarmacy.com). It is so pure that instead of being hard granules, it is as fine as a powder dust. It is super-salty and tastes much "cleaner" than regular table salt. I did an interesting experiment. I washed and polished two clear drinking glasses. I filled them both half full with distilled water. I added two tablespoons of table salt to one and two tablespoons of my raw salt to the other. I let the glasses sit in a sunny window sill for a couple of weeks. As the water evaporated, I could clearly see an almost milky residue on the sides of the table salt glass. After all of the water evaporated, my raw salt glass was perfectly clear except for the powder-like salt left at the bottom of the glass. The other glass had residue all the way from the original water line to the bottom of the glass where a hard-crystalline salt residue was left. Although the glass was not clear, it was clear to me that there were things other than salt in the table salt glass. This experiment proved the worth of pure salt to me.

My body loves and craves salt. I come from a family where both sides of my gene pool have heart and high blood pressure problems. I am happy to say that my blood pressure has always been perfect for all of my annual check-ups.

Keep salt in your diet in moderation - just purchase the purest, cleanest form possible.

Got Muck?

Dairy PRODUCTS ARE SUPPOSED TO be one of the four basic food groups – right? Hmmm...

Food for thought: Who was the first person to drink cow's milk? Did one cave man dare another to do it? Did a bunch of cow-tipping pranksters decide to take things to another level? Would you crawl under a cow, and squeeze a nipple directly into your mouth? Of course not – that's "utterly" disgusting - it has to be pasteurized and chilled in the fridge, right? A friend of mine worked at a dairy farm briefly and told me that not only did they pasteurize milk to get out harmful bacteria, but there was also a bleaching process involved because the milk was orange from blood in the milk because the cows were mechanically milked by machines until they bled. Not to mention all of the antibiotics and steroids given to the cows to make them produce more milk which all end up in the milk.

The only animal meant to naturally drink cow's milk is a baby cow. Cows don't even drink cow's milk once they are weaned. Humans are meant to drink their mother's breast milk until they are weaned and can eat solid food. Humans are the only animal that will willingly drink another animal's milk and we are also the only animals to drink milk after we are weaned.

If you suffer from allergies, try cutting dairy products from your diet. Dairy products stimulate the release of histamines in the body which can exacerbate the effects of pollen, pet dander and other allergens on your body's defense system.

Another common misconception is that milk is a great source of calcium. Granted, milk does contain calcium. However, ingesting cow's milk does not benefit the human body with calcium. In fact, it is my belief that drinking milk actually causes us to lose calcium. How? Think about this. What if digesting cow's milk caused your body's digestive system to burn massive amounts of energy to process and eliminate the milk and its' by-products. Furthermore, what if the digestion and breakdown of milk and dairy products in our digestive system caused acidic toxins to be released into our bodies? What if our body defended itself by leaching an alkaline substance such as calcium from our bones to combat the acidic toxins? What a paradox – we drink milk for calcium, but the digestion of milk causes a net loss of calcium.

I used to absolutely love cheese. Even after I became a vegetarian I still indulged in cheese for a while. I went to a health seminar shortly thereafter and changed my mind about cheese. Have you ever cooked a piece of pizza and had some cheese run out onto the pan? You scoop it up with your finger while it is hot and suck the soft, stringy, sticky gooey cheese down your hatch. Now think about the glob of cheese you didn't scoop off of the pan while it was still hot. You return to the kitchen later to wash dishes and find that the cheese is no longer soft, stringy, sticky and gooey – it is hard as a rock and you have to chisel it off of the pan. Now imagine the same process happening in your body. The problem in our long, narrow, winding intestines is two-fold. Everyone knows that eating too much cheese can "clog you up" and constipate you, thus preventing waste from leaving the body and causing a build-up of toxins. Not only does it clog you up, but it also leaves a residue on the lining of your intestines. This lining of gooey and hardening cheese will cause your intestines to not be able to absorb the nutrients from the good food that you eat. So, in essence, it clogs you up in more ways than one by not letting the bad stuff out of your body and not letting the good stuff get absorbed.

I've heard that it is estimated that the average American has 15 pounds of waste constantly impacted in their bowels. Do you work out and do sit-ups constantly, but just can't seem to get rid of the little pouch in your gut? Try water fasting, a raw food detox or a colon cleansing enema - and cut the cheese! I know it sounds like a "pain in the ass", but it just may save your ass!

Think Fast

IT IS MY PERSONAL BELIEF that fasting is a very healthy thing to do. The human body is designed to go for periods of time with no food. Long before grocery stores and restaurants, man had to grow, harvest and hunt for his food. There were periods of time during drought, famine and winter where food was not readily available every day or even every week. So man had to be able to go without food from time to time. Many other animals can also go very long periods of time – even whole seasons without any food. A bear hibernates all winter without eating. You may be thinking that a bear is very fat and has a lot of food stored away for the long winter fast, but what about a snake? Certain snakes can go for extended periods of time without food even when it is not hibernating. Man is also capable of this, but our bodies have become so programmed and spoiled that we anticipate a certain portion of food at certain times every day. It may be mentally and physically challenging at first, but you can have the ability to re-program your body, break your eating cycle and transition into a fasting period.

I once read an interesting article about research done on some of the largest living things on earth – trees. Researchers grew oak trees in a controlled environment. The amount of soil in each pot was weighed right down to the fraction of a gram and the water content of the soil was calculated and the seed was also weighed. The only thing added to the soil during the growth of the tree was mineral rich water and the only other ingredients given to the tree was air and sunlight. Years later when the oak tree had grown into a substantial sapling, it was removed from the soil in its entirety. Every speck of soil was dusted and washed off of the tree roots. The soil was then weighed and the moisture content was calculated so that water weight could be factored in. Guess what – there was exactly the same amount of soil – right down to the gram that there was in the pot to start with. An oak tree weighing over 50 pounds was grown in soil and given only water, sunlight and air. Nothing was taken from the soil. Only the nutrients in the water and the carbon in the air contributed to the tree's mass. Ironically, trees and plants can grow to massive sizes and take nothing from the soil other than nutrient rich water, but plants and trees contribute to the soil when their foliage falls to the ground and decomposes into compost.

Further proof that trees and plants can grow with only nutrient rich water is evident in hydroponic farming. I did an experiment of my own to test the nutrient rich water theory. I bought two bamboo sprouts of equal size in glass vases with only glass marbles in the bottom. I filled one with municipal tap water and one with mineral rich FIJI water. I grew the two bamboo shoots in the same environment with the same air, temperature and sunlight exposure. Within a year the FIJI plant had outgrown the tap water plant. Within two years, the FIJI plant was three times the size of the tap water plant and was much greener and had healthy leaves. Within three years, the tap water plant had yellowed and died. Five years later, the FIJI plant is still thriving and is healthy and green. Was it a coincidence? Did I just have a sick bamboo plant to start with that would have died even if I had given it FIJI water? Well, I admit that there were only two plants and that my test did not involve thorough scientific research and control values. However, both plants looked identical to start with and they were both exposed to the same things – with the exception of the water. When I dumped out the dead bamboo shoot, I noticed the vase and marbles were covered and stained with a reddish residue. I recognized the same red residue forming a ring inside my toilet bowl if I went on vacation or didn't clean it for a while. I did a little research and found out that it was from the fluoride in the city tap water. That's pretty scary - because fluoride is highly toxic even though it is touted for its dental attributes. I prefer to avoid intentionally putting known toxins into my body regardless of what positive attributes they 'supposedly' have. I would rather rely on Mother Nature to provide me the natural minerals and nutrients in my water.

The largest normal energy drain on the body is its own digestive process. That's why it is common to get very tired and lethargic after eating a large meal. In fact, many people get the urge to take an afternoon nap right after lunch every day. Your body is using massive amounts of energy to digest the meal you just ate and it doesn't have energy left to carry out other activities. Not only is your body using massive amounts of energy to digest cooked food, but the digestion is also depleting your body's enzyme bank that is used to break down the food. Cooking kills the enzymes in food. When you eat raw food, your body is able to use the living enzymes in the raw food to aid in the digestive process while not taxing your enzyme reserve. Metabolic energy can be diverted from digestion during strenuous activity such as running, swimming or even sex. But when the body has nothing to digest, it has the ability to temporarily shut down the digestive system and divert the energy to the brain and other organs. This energy diversion from digestion to the other organs gives the body a chance to do a little "house cleaning". This house cleaning can lead to great detoxification of the internal organs and even the skin.

When your body is hungry it goes into survival mode. Your brain kicks into high gear and instincts take over. You become more focused and alert and in touch with your surroundings. It is this instinct that helped drive our ancestors to survive when times were tough and going to get food involved more than driving to the store.

Fasting can take your body to its ideal weight. The time frame depends on how deep in the hole you start and how overweight or underweight you are. During a fast, your body burns stored fat and releases toxins that were trapped within the fat. Drinking copious amounts of water during the fasting period will ensure that these toxins are properly eliminated from the body.

A "fast" is a fast way to lose weight and detoxify. Start out with baby steps and challenge yourself to go 36 hours with only water - lots of water. After your 36 hours of water, try to go another 36 hours with only fresh juice such as wheatgrass, carrot, apple or CABALA. This water/juice fast will cause your body to detoxify and many toxins will end up in your colon ready for elimination. It is important to sweep the colon out and further clean house. I use what I call a "colon sweep salad". Here is the recipe: Shredded carrots, grated beets, grated red cabbage, chopped celery and then squeeze a fresh orange on top for salad dressing. Eat this salad three times a day for two or three days and your colon will be swept clean. This thorough sweeping will remove impacted waste and embedded toxins in the colon and clear the way for nutrient absorption. When the colon is clean, the body will operate much more efficiently and body odors will be greatly reduced. Almost all body odors originate and emanate from the colon - when it is clean, the rest of your body will benefit too.

Once you have fasted on water and juice and then swept your colon clean you have paved the way for weight loss and detoxification to begin. The shock of the fast to your digestive system should make the reprogramming process easier now. Immediately following the colon sweep begin a raw food diet. This raw food diet should consist of 6 to 8 meals a day of raw, fresh, organic fruits and vegetables - the greener the better. Citrus fruits and berries are ideal for breakfast followed by a banana for a mid-morning snack. A shot of wheatgrass juice in the morning instead of coffee is great too. Indulge in a huge salad for lunch - make it green and colorful, skip the cheese, egg and other non-raw items and add olive oil for salad dressing. Eat an avocado or an apple for an afternoon snack. Enjoy a glass of fresh carrot juice for a late afternoon pick-me-up. Have another large salad at least 4 hours before bedtime to finish off the day's eating. Continue this raw food eating and watch the pounds melt off, your hair and skin become healthier and your energy levels and concentration increase.

It is the preceding advice that led me to a predominantly vegetarian and raw food diet over a decade ago. It is the healthy feeling and the disease free life that has motivated me to stay on that wagon. Many friends and people I know have started out strong on this new way of eating and have had some immediate and profound positive results, but have reverted back to old habits and undone all of their progress. Countless people have asked me "So if I do this fast and raw food diet for a month and lose weight, will I gain it back after I stop eating raw?" Common sense dictates that if you revert back to the old habits that put the weight on you in the first place that it will certainly come back again. Let feeling healthy and looking great outweigh the temptations of your former self.

Yoga, stretching, sauna, deep breathing, good posture and LOTS OF WATER are essential partners in the fasting process.

Polluted Population

MY DEFINITION OF POLLUTION IS "anything detrimental introduced into an otherwise clean, stable and healthy environment". Pollution is everywhere and it is both man-made and naturally occurring. The naturally occurring pollution is usually absorbed and cleansed by natural processes while the man-made pollution can be resistant and harmful to nature. For instance, animal feces or dead organic matter goes through a natural decomposition process and ultimately returns to nature as organic matter. In fact, these organic waste products act as food on which other organisms thrive as they do their job as natural recyclers. On the other hand, plastics, Styrofoam, textiles and other man-made products can linger in nature indefinitely and are impervious to natural decomposition processes.

Pollution doesn't have to necessarily be anything tangible such as gas, liquid or solids. It can also be in the form of noise. Noise pollution can initiate stress and be very detrimental to mental health. If you have ever lived near a construction zone or had a neighbor with an erratic car alarm, then you know what I am talking about. Noise can kill peace and quiet and mental tranquility in an instant.

People can also inadvertently contribute to pollution in their own houses without knowing it. One of the worst domestic pollutants is dust and the largest contributors of dust particles are human and animal dander. Dander is formed when animals shed their dead skin cells and hair. These cells become airborne in our homes, cars and offices. Dust mites, mold, fungus and other parasites feed on these dead cells. We then breathe this polluted air into our lungs and introduce these intruders into a very comfortable environment for them to continue to thrive and breed – at our expense. Our body retaliates and tries to rid itself of these intruders with cold and flu-like symptoms. Bathing ourselves and our pets in clean, pure water with natural soaps and shampoos and using organic lotions on our skin can help reduce dander.

The best way to fight this domestic pollution is to stop it before it gets into our bodies. Keeping a clean house, car and workspace is the best place to start. But before you go grabbing your vacuum cleaner, be advised that vacuuming often worsens the problem of airborne pollutants. The average vacuum cleaner just sucks up the big, visible stuff but redistributes the small and most harmful particles back into the air. A true HEPA filter vacuum cleaner will minimize recirculation of dust particles down to the smallest microns and keep your air clean while you suck up the dust and dirt.

Another great dust fighting tool is an air filter in your home. Almost all housing that has a central air A/C and heat system has an air filter in it. If you don't have a central air system (you may have radiators for heat and window units for A/C) then you can purchase a stand-alone air filter at almost any department store. This air filter needs changing at least once every three months. Use of a HEPA or small-micron filter will cost a little extra, but will benefit you by doing what an air filter was really meant to do. Changing the filter regularly will save energy and prolong the life of your central air unit or air filtration system by easing the flow of air and reducing the stress on the fan. Adding an ultra violet light or ionizer to your central air system or air filter will also kill mold and bacteria that may circumvent the filter. I have been using an ionizer in my home for the last 10 years and I have seen a remarkable difference in my allergies and frequency of illness. An ionizer acts as an invisible cleanser by negatively charging the particles in the air and causing them to ground themselves. This grounding effect keeps particulate on the ground and surfaces where they are easily visible and cleaned up and not in the air you breathe. The same ionization effect is evident in nature after a thunderstorm. The immense energy released by lightning in the air ionizes the air which forms ozone. This ozone causes particulate in the air to become negatively charged and grounded. These particles are then washed away by rain water. That is why the air seems so clean and crisp after a thunderstorm.

More man-made pollution is all around us every day in the form of radio waves. Think about all of the radio frequencies, cell phones, satellite signals, microwaves, wireless devices and even car door and garage door openers that are in use every second of every day. If you could wear special glasses that would expose these radio waves, I doubt you would be able to see your hand in front of your face from all of the interference and energy in the air. How detrimental is this radio pollution to our health? Who knows?! Much of this technology is too new to have long term test results. Common sense would dictate that it can't be healthy since it wasn't meant to be penetrating our bodies. Maybe that has something to do with the outrageous cancer incidence in our industrialized and technology rich society.

Do your part to minimize pollution. If everyone makes small changes, it will lead to big results. Walk, run or bike – it will cut out harmful carbon emissions from exhaust fumes while burning calories and fat in our bodies. Reducing the use of automobiles will also cut down on traffic, wear and tear on roadways, oil dependency, car maintenance, tire replacement, chance of accidents, DUI's and traffic violations. Another way to conserve is to limit phone conversations - be brief and to the point. This will not only cut down your phone bill, but will also cut down on radio waves and energy used by your battery and energy used to recharge your battery. You can also conserve while shopping. Buy textiles that are made from organic substances such as cotton or silk and try to buy garments that do not require dry cleaning (another huge pollutant). Wash your garments in environmentally friendly organic detergents.

We only have one body and one planet. We need to respect both and do our part to keep them clean and safe. Future generations are counting on us to do our part now to insure the future environment will be clean and life supporting.

A Breath of Fresh Air

ONCE YOU HAVE CLEANED AND escaped the pollution, take a deep breath of clean fresh air and see how invigorating it can be. Focus on your posture and breath. Notice how much deeper you can breathe when sitting or standing up straight. When you hunch over or slouch, you are not allowing the lungs to fill to their full capacity. You are essentially suffocating the body with hunched back and short breaths. When you take deep, conscious breaths you bring oxygen deep into the lungs and blood. This fully oxygenated blood fuels the body's cells more rapidly and can increase energy, resilience and disease resistance. Scientific research suggests that cancer can't survive in oxygen rich environments. Deeper breathing coupled with inversion exercises can cure headaches and relieve sleeplessness. Yawning could be cited as an instinctual reaction to the body's need for more oxygen. Yoga gives excellent practice in taking full breaths and combining breathing with body motion.

What to Do

- Think positive thoughts and smile as much as possible – even in the face of adversity

- Join a gym that is convenient, clean and full of features and people that will help motivate you to go there.

- Do a water fast for at least 72 hours

- Complete a 14 day raw food and juice detoxification and make every attempt to cut out future consumption of artificial substances.

- Set some challenging yet attainable personal goals and write them down

- Break bad habits and replace them with good ones

- Find a health food supplement that is right for you – visit the Health and Happiness/Healthy business section on SeanDon. com for some great recommendations.

- Reduce your stress through stretching, relaxation and meditation or take a vacation.

- Drink lots of pure, mineral rich water and add a good home water filtration/purification system to help take harmful substances out of the tap water that you bathe and wash dishes and clothes in.

- Keep your body, home, car and workplace clean. Bathe in pure filtered water and use natural soaps and cosmetics. Install an air filtration and ionization system in your home.

- Keep an open mind and review all ideas logically with your own common sense.

- Appreciate your fortunes, no matter how small or insignificant they may seem.

- Learn from misfortunes and the mistakes that you and others around you will undoubtedly make.

- Walk as much as possible.

- Stop procrastinating – tomorrow may never come – focus on today.

- Don't worry and stress about things you have no control over – concentrate positive energy on things you can control and influence - starting with your attitude.

- Pass some good advice along to someone who may need it – share this book and website with friends and family.

- Buy locally grown organic produce.

- If you must eat meat, buy meat that was raised naturally without antibiotics and growth hormones from animals that were raised in nature, not cages.

- Read your goals list daily and track your accomplishments

- Also check out the "Healthy Business" section of Seandon. com

- Exercise:

Exercise

MAKE LITTLE CHANGES IN YOUR life to burn a few extra calories.

- Park at the back of parking lots and walk a few extra steps.

- Take the stairs instead of elevators

- Walk your dog

- If you have a desk job which requires you to sit at a workstation, stand up for at least 5 minutes per hour and stretch. It will make your other 55 minutes per hour at the desk more relaxed, productive and less stressful.

- Take a few minutes each hour or so to do some heel to toe rebound exercises.

- Buy a small 36" rebound trampoline and jump for 20 minutes daily.

- Join a gym – it's a great way to make new friends and network your business while getting in shape.

- Practice yoga at home

- Do sit-ups at home while watching TV or do leg-lifts while sitting on the couch

- Stretch and "Flexercise" while driving or sitting at your desk at work

- Induce sweat with exercise or sauna

Sean's Words of Wisdom

1. Follow the Golden Rule – "Do unto others as you would have them do unto you"

2. Make every minute of every day productive in some kind of way.

3. A day spent upset is a day you might regret. You only get one life to live - you better make it positive. So turn a frown upside down and smile for a while.

4. Focus on what you can control first and then things previously out of control will fall into place. Start with your attitude because it is the only thing that you truly have 100% control over.

5. Realize that your attitude is based on your perception of things. Your perception of things can be skewed depending on the "angle" at which you look at the particular thing. Change your angle and change your perception and your attitude will follow.

6. Always leave things (and people) better than you found them.

7. Speak only the truth and you will never have to remember anything.

8. Inaction is the best recipe for failure and mediocrity.

9. Your body is your temple, worship it.

10. Without health everything else is irrelevant.

11. You only live once, so do it right.

12. What goes around comes around and Karma is the great equalizer.

13. Strive for perfection, but settle only for your best.

14. When life gives you 100 reasons to cry, show life 1000 reasons to smile.

15. Beat the unbeaten path.

16. True wealth is in the heart and mind, not the pocket or the bank.

17. There is no such thing as a bad day, only a better one.

18. Happy is how you should live - so try to focus on being positive.

19. Live every day as if you should have died yesterday.

20. He who dies with the biggest smile wins.

21. It's not the clothes, jewelry, makeup or hair, but the look on your face that matters most.

22. Your body is your house – keep it clean and healthy.

23. Life is a game, just like any game there are winners and losers. The winners are the ones that know how to play the game and make their own rules as they go. The losers allow life to manipulate them and dictate the rules. Losers simply react. The winners get out and live life. Winners have few regrets. They know how to turn negative situations into positive ones. They are the "glass is half full" people. The winners are the

ones you see in the supermarket smiling. The losers are always unhappy, complaining about trivial nothings. They do not realize that life is precious – that you only get one shot.

24. Everyone makes mistakes in life. The winners learn from their mistakes and do not make the same ones again. Every mistake is a learning experience. The losers dwell on their mistakes and tend to make the same ones again and again. Like a bad movie, they replay them in their head over and over again. Get over it and move on. If you rent a bad movie at the video store, you don't go back and rent it again. Forget about it – look forward to knowing that you will never do THAT again!

25. There is only one now. There will never be another exact moment in time like now. Cherish the now. Don't waste time. Make every moment of every day productive and positive.

26. If you have to do something, you might as well make it enjoyable.

27. "An eye for an eye" attitude will make the world go blind.

28. It's not how old you are, but how old you look, feel and act that matters.

29. The trivial things don't really amount to much in the whole scheme of things. Don't dwell on them – concentrate on the finer and more important things in life.

30. Time is only relative to what you compare it to. In some instances, an hour can seem like an eternity – like sitting in traffic after a long day at work. However, an hour of incredible sex can fly by in seconds. Think about the best hour of your life and live it over and over again when you find yourself in a bad situation. You may be amazed at how quickly the bad situation will pass. Use you "hour of power" as constant motivation every day. Relive the hour and recall all of the sensory perceptions associated with it. Put yourself back in that hour on command at any time you may need a positive

lift. Learn to control your attitude and emotions in all states of mind.

31. If you don't expect the best you may never be let down, but you may never accomplish your best. Do your best all of the time and you will exceed your own wildest expectations. If you fail, you fail. Learn from it and find something that you can do better. Or find another way to do the thing that you failed at.

32. It's not how much you make that matters, it's what you keep that counts.

33. If you wake up and put two feet on the ground – it's going to be a good day.

34. A challenge is your opportunity to step up and do your best – SHINE.

35. To err is human – to forgive is divine. Start by forgiving yourself.

36. If you think things can't get any worse, you'd be surprised how wrong you are.

37. It's hard to smile when you are upset, but it is hard to be upset when you are smiling. So turn your frown upside down and smile for a while.

38. What's right to one may be wrong to another. It's all in how you interpret it. Refer to item #1 and live by the Golden Rule and do unto others as you would have them do unto you

39. "Dream as if you will live forever and live as if you will die today" - (James Dean)

I'll Rest When I Die
A Tribute to NA

THERE WAS A WOMAN VERY close to me who inspired me to live life to its fullest. She was my "grand" mother for 31 years of my life. During those years, I witnessed a lifetime of love and righteous living that few people could ever have the pleasure of experiencing or even envisioning. She left me an inheritance more valuable than a million dollar estate. In return, I affectionately named her "Na" and I will cherish her in my heart and memories for ever and share her story with those who need inspiration.

She was my closest family member to pass away, save her sister, my saint-like Aunt Lucy who I now refer to as my guardian angel. As sad as it was to lose someone so close to me I found solace in the fact that she had everything "in order" when she died. She had no last minute apologies, no regrets, no ambiguity and most importantly, no guilt. No loose ends were left untied. I believe that Na could have passed away at any time and not left a burden behind for anyone to contend with. True to form as the great housekeeper she was, she kept her life neat and in order as well. She had her bags packed and ready to go whenever the Lord was ready for her.

Na was full of intuition and premonition all of her life. She always knew when something was wrong or when someone was about to call or visit. How ironic that she knew it was her own time to go upon checking in to the hospital for abdominal pains. She blessed me by passing her sixth sense along to me starting the instant she died. I'll never forget the moment when I realized it. It was a sunny day in Virginia Beach and I was driving my boat with my brother to take my mind off of the fact that Na was in the intensive care unit at the hospital. I had already said my goodbyes to her the day before as I knew that she would be taken off of life support at her request today. I bent over to grab my water bottle which was rolling across the deck of my boat and I hit my sunglasses on the metal windshield frame. The corner of the frame caused a small scratch on the polarized lens of my glasses allowing a ray of unfiltered light to shine through. Before I could formulate a thought about the scratch, my phone rang. When I saw it was my mom on the caller ID, I didn't even have to hear the sorrow in her voice before I knew Na had passed. That ray of light a second beforehand was her signaling me from heaven. Since that moment I have experienced a new awareness in my life.

At age 89 Na had the health and mobility of the average 60 year old in this country. An amazing feat, considering she had been through 2 hip replacement surgeries and a colon removal. A lot of people wouldn't have survived what she lived through - they would have given up and been bed-ridden 10, 20, 40 years prior. A friend of mine went with me to my grandparent's house for a visit one afternoon. She was awestruck to see my grandma on hands and knees scrubbing the kitchen floor – because she knew how old she was and knew what she had been through! I was shocked when I heard from my uncle that they were taking Na to the hospital because just the week before I had witnessed her cleaning the house and cooking. Her words still resound in my memories today "you've got to keep doing until you die - or you will die" she would say to me. There is no doubt in my mind that her daily and weekly routine and devout adherence to those is what kept her healthy and alive for so long.

With the exception of drinking governmentally-polluted well water for a large portion of her life, Na lived a very healthy and active lifestyle. She did not own a microwave and wouldn't have thought of using one if she did. No sir, all meals were home-cooked the old fashioned way with natural ingredients and love. She would put out holiday meal spreads that would rival the work of a team of souse chefs and she would do it by herself in a humble kitchen with a standard 30" electric stove. This feat would be difficult or even impossible for anyone her age, but she did it with a smile and made it look easy. I once had a vision of her as a little girl watching her mother cook not a holiday meal, but a nightly meal in a country style kitchen with a wood stove and no running water. I then knew why Na cooked with a smile – her kitchen was heaven to her - a girlhood fantasy inconceivable in her era and state of technology at that time. It was this realization that afforded me a viable argument to a contractor who was putting me off on some trim work on a historic renovation of a house I owned. After 2 weeks of lollygagging, he told me that he didn't have the right nail gun to do the job. I know the construction of late nineteenth century houses and I know that when the houses were originally built they didn't have any nail guns - in fact, they were lucky to get a straight nail from the blacksmith. It was apparent to me that this guy didn't have the will power to work at age 25. I thought about my Na cooking in her kitchen every day, 3 times a day for her and my grandfather and occasional guests. She never missed having a double oven or a microwave; she made it work with what she had. She resisted the urge for take-out or prepared foods or frozen microwave meals. She avoided the easy way out. She never missed things that a lot of people take for granted today.

Na was cultured deeply in her own way. It blew my mind that she never experienced Italian or Mexican food. "Spicy things didn't agree with her" she would say. What she did experience was the wholesome goodness of home-made (and home-grown in many instances) food that she made with love. I swear she made the best tasting meal you could ever eat. Home baked rolls, corn-puddin', fried okra, butterbeans, snaps and cobbler with special sugar sauce were some of her specialties. I would pay 5 star dining prices for one of her meals any day.

Their back yard garden yielded an abundance of organic goodness which they lovingly shared with family, friends and neighbors. My grandfather (Da) would drive through the quiet neighborhood on his tractor pulling a trailer full of fresh fruits and veggies and would dole them out to everyone he knew. Na's grapevine was the envy of every bird for miles. Even after sharing with everyone and the birds too, somehow there was always enough left over for canning and preserving. It was almost like Jesus sharing the fish. There was always enough to share and for them sharing came first. Na would give you the shirt off of her back, or better yet, make you one of your own. As a child I watched in perplexity as the bobbin on her Singer sewing machine plunged in and out of a piece of fabric taught between her fingers with careful calculation and precision. Her concentration was amazing and her handy-work was typically flawless with a certain degree of

"Na-ness" or love sewn in to every fiber. I was teased as a kid by classmates for some of the home-made fashion I wore, but looking back, I know they were only jealous that their grandmother either lacked the life, time, ability or most importantly desire to craft such a garment for them. Was it her time in the "spool room" working the looms which produced fibers for DuPont that taught her this skill or was it inherited from her mother or self taught? Either way, most people probably wouldn't want to even see a needle and thread if they worked in a post-depression factory doing the same thing hours on end every shift-work week. She took the skill to a different level and never accepted a penny for any of her button sewing or hemming services for friends and family.

I don't think Na would want anyone to be sad about her death. I think I am a lot like her and I think we both share the same view on post life wishes. She led by example and I think the highest compliment that I can give her is to emulate her in certain ways. Times have changed drastically since she was my age, but certain values and morals are timeless. She taught me that the most important thing you can leave behind to a loved one or the good of the people is a great impression. Have you known anyone for 31 years? Could you look back and honestly remember them never complaining about anything, or bad mouthing anyone, or fighting with their spouse, or speaking of some ailment that you know they have? Even when times were probably tough, you would never guess it from meeting her. She loved her husband with benevolent devotion till death did part them. Together they made a perfect team. Na had her "software" chores and routines in the house and garden and Da handled the "hardware" side of things in the garage. They were the Yen and the Yang of life.

Although I am not a devout Christian like Na, she taught me that you should believe in something whether it is religion or simply believing in yourself. Without a higher belief, the mind becomes stale and the heart loses hope. A higher belief keeps you ascending higher in life and gives you purpose, morals, values, history and discipline. I wonder how many times she read the Bible before going to sleep at night. She believed and prayed daily and always practiced what she preached. She truly walked the walk.

Na was a grandmother, a mother, a role model and a friend to me all of my life. She made my childhood special with her "goodie bags" that she would prepare for me and my brother (but only after we ate our veggies). To this day my mouth waters when I glimpse that left-hand door of the buffet in the dining room where she used to keep the sweets. Junior mints, candy bars and all kinds of treats resided in there - it was like a candy store! Not only did their quaint Cape Cod house appeal to my sweet tooth as a child, but also had the aura of a carnival fun-house. I'll never forget the adventure of following Na into the storage eaves on the second floor that she nicknamed "man-holes". She made such an adventure out of something as simple as looking for yarn in storage. There were always some cool antique toys or other keepsakes to be found in there. No matter how busy Na was with her own tasks and chores, she never hesitated a moment to go out of her way to make sure my brother and I were entertained, fed and comfortable.

Na was a spendthrift with her love, but frugal in every other aspect. I watched her wash Saran wrap and Aluminum foil and spread it on the counter to dry for reuse later. I saw her pour salt and pepper packets from take-out restaurants into her shakers at home. I thought surely my grandparents could afford to buy salt and pepper – after all, they paid off their house in only seven years. Then I realized that it was frugality like that which allowed them to pay off their house so soon when other families remained married to a 30 year mortgage. Living through the great depression taught them the value of a dollar (or a nickel in those times).

Every aspect of Na and Da remained as constant and stable as the sunrise in the east. From the décor in their house, the beautiful blooming Dogwoods and John-quills in their yard in the spring, the summer vegetable garden, the Concord grapevine, the smell of her rolls in the oven, Baptist Church Sunday morning and the Chesterfield airport restaurant Sunday lunch buffet to grocery shopping on Thursdays – her routine was clockwork. Her daily routine translated into yearly holiday traditions as well. You could always count on a comfortable, loving family environment and a home-cooked meal every Christmas, Thanksgiving and birthday. She and Da always put the extra touch on the holiday to make it special. I will never forget the Christmas wonderland that the basement transformed into with the antique Christmas lights and the pile of neatly wrapped presents covering the washer and dryer in the corner. My favorite Christmas tradition of all was the "Boom-Bag". It was a Na-made red naga-hyde bag with a broom stick handle at the top and a draw string at the bottom. She and Da would pack it full of every goodie and trinket imaginable and they would even stuff some cash in some unsuspecting tissue packet or something. The entire family would sit in a circle in the floor as Na and Da held the bag high overhead. When she pulled that draw string, a pile of joy fell onto the floor and the whole family delved in for their share. You could only use one hand - the other hand held your own plastic bag - and it wasn't yours until it was in your bag! When the looting was done, we would all sit around the table and check out our bounty and trade between ourselves. What a cool tradition.

Na would defend and "rescue" me sometimes when Da would pick on me. I will never forget when Da generously offered to give me his 1972 Ford LTD "greenie" when I turned 16. Na, in her infinite wisdom, said "Jake, he doesn't want that big old car, he wants something sporty". She couldn't have been more right, but I would have never had the heart to tell it to Da. Na always knew when something was bothering me and she always knew how to make it better. She was in tune with everything and everyone around her.

The best way for me to honor Na is to carry her memories fresh in my mind and live life to the fullest as she did. She used to console me when I was distraught because my younger brother was "copying me". She would tell me that "imitation is the highest form of flattery." She has inspired me to "copy" and imitate her in many ways. I have expensive taste and will never be frugal like her, but I conserve and recycle whenever possible. She taught me that helping others can bring a great sense of accomplishment and that generosity will be rewarded tenfold. I gained a green thumb and affection for gardening because of her and I now take great pride in growing my own herbs and adorning my house and yard with plants in the spring and summer. I clean my house with energy and a smile instead of disdain. I always appreciate a home cooked meal and the love, time and energy that goes into cooking one. Every time my mother cooks some rolls or corn-pudding, I thank my grandmother for teaching her those skills. I witnessed a wonderful 70 year long marriage between her and Da and aspire to have the same situation myself and I know that it will work if I have the same respect for my wife that Na and Da had for each other. I will have children one day and will endure the same patience that Na had with me and my brother. I will go out of my way to make every occasion special for my friends and family. I miss Na always, but will always remember and cherish the memories and examples that she left behind. I will continue her legacy and traditions by passing them on to my family and friends in the future.

Rest in peace, Na – and know that you are loved and remembered by those whom you loved.

What do you Think?

NOW THAT I HAVE SHARED my thoughts and ideas with you, please do the same in return. I would love to hear your opinion on my Health and Happiness Guide. Please forward all comments and/or constructive criticism to sean@seandon.com. I greatly appreciate the feedback.

About the Author

SEAN "SEANDON" DONOVAN HAS BEEN passionately writing since the second grade. He writes non-fiction, novels, "fictitious reality", shorts and poems - about whatever happens to be on his mind at the time. His passion for writing is fueled by the fact that writing is something that the author has complete control over. The author controls the characters, the attitudes, the tone and the outcome of his stories. Sean's philosophy is that aside from your attitude and your writing, there are not many things in life that you can completely control. He also believes that the pen truly is mightier than the sword and "writing wrongs" is a great way to deal with adversity and problems in your life. Writing can also be done anytime, anywhere - with a digital recorder, laptop or good ol' fashioned pen and paper. As an avid traveler, Sean has done some of his best writing while traveling. He finds inspiration for his writing in the people he meets and different places and cultures he has visited.

Although Sean never intended to write for profit (only fun), a downturn in the economy shifted him away from his primary business in Real Estate and Contracting and motivated him to do what he really loves - writing. Sean realized that art in the form of music, painting, drawing and writing is one of the most profound things you can share with the public. Art is a great way to express yourself, influence others and leave a piece of your mind behind for others to enjoy once you are gone.

Sean believes that knowledge is power and every day is an opportunity to learn something new. After reading dozens and dozens of health related books, conducting extensive research on the internet, attending numerous health seminars, emulating other healthy people and experimenting with his own diet and exercise routine, Sean has become an expert in health and happiness.

Sean's first published book "Health and Happiness" is a compilation of good, common sense advice for healthy, happy living. Over a decade of being a positive person, a vegetarian and raw food advocate has afforded him a disease free lifestyle and has helped him avoid hereditary health problems in his family. Sean led by example and became the go-to guy for friends who were having both health problems and emotional stress. He began writing down the advice he was giving to others and, before he knew it, he had compiled a couple hundred pages of great advice based on his own experiences. Inspired by friends, the current state of the health care system and the loss of several people dear to him, he decided to condense his advice into an easy to read book in hopes that he may help many other people find "Health and Happiness" in their lives.

www.ingramcontent.com/pod-product-compliance
Lightning Source LLC
Chambersburg PA
CBHW022255290526
45785CB00015B/1008